SKIN CAMOUFLAGE

A Guide to Remedial Techniques

Victoria – Dallas
1995

Also by Stanley Thornes (Publishers) Ltd

Elaine Almond	*Safety in the Salon*
W E Arnould-Taylor	*The Principles and Practice of Physical Therapy*
W E Arnould-Taylor	*Aromatherapy for the Whole Person*
Ann Gallant	*Body Treatments and Dietetics for the Beauty Therapist*
Ann Gallant	*Principles and Techniques for the Electrologist*
Ann Gallant	*Principles and Techniques for the Beauty Specialist*
Ann Hagman	*The Aestheticienne*
John Rounce	*Science for the Beauty Therapist*

Beauty Guides by Ann Gallant

1 Muscle Contraction Treatment
2 Figure Treatment
3 Galvanic Treatment
4 Epilation Treatment

Skin Camouflage

A Guide to Remedial Techniques

Joyce Allsworth

Stanley Thornes (Publishers) Ltd

First published in 1985 by
Stanley Thornes (Publishers) Ltd,
Old Station Drive,
Leckhampton,
CHELTENHAM GL53 0DN

British Library Cataloguing in Publication Data

Allsworth, Joyce
    Skin camouflage: a guide to remedial techniques
    1. Skin—Abnormalities
    2. Skin—Wounds and injuries
    3. Cosmetics
    I. Title
    646.7'26   RL87

ISBN 0-85950-151-5

Typeset in 10/12 Garamond
by Tech-Set, Gateshead, Tyne & Wear.
Printed and bound in Great Britain
at The Bath Press, Avon.

Contents

Foreword

People are aware of their own appearance and the reactions of others to it. To be attractive is all that some require. To be attractive is important to others. Mirrors and photographs allow us to be seen as others see us. Comments are made and questions are asked about our appearance, even when we are perfectly normal. If we are born abnormal or made abnormal by accident, or disease, the focus of our own or other's attention may be on the abnormality and so obstructive that the abnormality cannot be forgotten.

For centuries, normal people have used dress, ornament, camouflage or cosmetics to alter the appearance of their bodies, to enhance the desirable, or to disguise or hide the unattractive aspects of their appearance. Vast sums of money are spent on clothing, ornaments and beauty care. Now, those who suffer some abnormality of appearance may be assisted by surgery to improve and sometimes resolve the problems.

Surgery, however, still has many shortcomings and although defects of contour, texture, colour and hairiness, resulting from disease or injury, may be improved by operation, there is often some residual imperfection.

For much of the time clothing will cover most of the body, but there are some areas such as the face and hands not normally covered. Other parts of the body must be uncovered in certain sporting or social activities. For such abnormalities cosmetic camouflage has much to offer.

This book deals with many examples of situations in which help can be given to assist patients to restore themselves to confidence in a normal appearance. Being written by an author with so much experience in the field of cosmetic camouflage, it may prove an invaluable aid to those who would wish to assist by teaching patients the invaluable techniques the book describes.

Cosmetic camouflage of abnormalities of appearance is as essential a part of restorative surgery as is the surgery itself. The contents of these pages contribute greatly to the propagation of available knowledge in this important field. They teach expertise, coupled with compassion, sympathy and optimistic realism, but thankfully without a trace of condescension. This book will help many with their need to be normal, and others to assist them to be so.

Roy Sanders BSc, MB, BS, FRCS
Consultant Plastic Surgeon

Preface

This book began some forty-two years ago. It was a wet summer afternoon during the war when two friends and I set off excitedly for London for a few hours away from our WAAF duties at North Weald, one of the now famous Battle of Britain RAF stations. We were lucky enough to hitch a ride in – of all things – a Rolls Royce, and the 16-mile journey to town was passed in high spirits. We chatted merrily to the driver, who, although he had lost his voice, seemed pleased to have met us and even offered us afternoon tea in a smart restaurant – this indeed was living! He took us to Frascati's, where the waiter produced a strawberry tea – a rare treat in those days.

I remember I was sitting facing the entrance in the vast room and suddenly became aware of a tall Air Force officer standing defiantly on the steps leading down towards me. He seemed to be commanding everyone to notice him and they did, because his face was a tortured mask. His nose, hair and eye-brows had been burned away leaving only his eyes and a ghastly twisted gap for his mouth. He looked like a scarcely covered skeleton; even his hands were red and claw-like.

I cannot adequately express in words the feeling of intense shock that his appearance gave me. Intense pity, revulsion and anger followed in quick succession. His looks personified all the human suffering I had ever seen. The rest of that day remains a blur, for at that moment I had realised the horror of war. The glamour I had associated with the 'boys in blue' was dulled and the cruelty of war became a reality which has never left me.

In sad moments during the following years I remembered that tortured face and assumed there were people who had helped him and others like him. In time I realised that it is not enough to feel sorrow and leave other people to pick up the pieces. We should all be prepared to become involved and make our own contribution.

After many years a dear friend gave me the confidence to do something myself. His words were, 'If you want something enough, then tell everyone you meet about it and in the end you will find someone who will help you achieve it'. It had taken decades for me to make my move, but I decided that from then on my aim must be to help disfigured people.

Eventually after training I was able to work alongside a marvellous surgeon who allowed me to learn and practise all that follows in this book.

As yet, there are not enough people doing camouflage work, so I hope this book will reach those who desperately need help themselves but as yet have been unable to find it. Other aims of this book are to promote more interest in cosmetic camouflage, to help schools give a more comprehensive training, and to those of you who have thought of taking up the work yourselves I hope it may bring further incentive and perhaps suggest more ways of achieving your ambition.

To the many people who have helped me to achieve my goal, I give my grateful thanks, especially to the surgeon who gave me my chance, but I dedicate this book to that unknown airman – wherever he may be.

Joyce Allsworth
1985

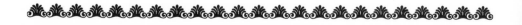

1

Introduction

Skin camouflage has until recently been one of the most neglected areas in therapeutic practice. But the hazards of modern life – the increase in traffic accidents, the effects of warfare – coupled with the growing unwillingness of society to accept visible scarring, have acted together to produce the need for treatment. As in other disciplines, individual practitioners and establishments have emerged to set the standards in the new skills. In the United Kingdom a great deal of pioneering work in this field was done at the Queen Victoria Hospital, East Grinstead, where many of the early patients were injured servicemen.

Scarring has many causes, ranging from birthmarks, vitiligo, chloasma and rosacea to surgery, road traffic accidents, burns, dog bites, surface thread veins and tribal markings. With skilled application of often simple routines, these conditions can be so improved as to bring substantial benefit to the patients. Indeed, camouflaging by properly applied creams can disguise or even obliterate most types of scarring.

With a growing awareness of the need for a treatment to disguise scarring, manufacturers of cosmetics have taken up the challenge and produced ranges of specifically designed cover creams. These differ from ordinary cosmetics in that they have greater covering qualities, are waterproof and resistant to the harmful ultra-violet rays of sunlight, and thus allow the wearer protection in every sense.

Scars will be presented for camouflage at many different stages. Some may have been present from birth or sustained in early life. In the case of fresh scars from trauma or surgery, it is desirable that these should be camouflaged as soon as possible, which in the case of surgery can be within a matter of days after the removal of the sutures. At this point the appearance is at its worst and the psychological effect is most damaging. Camouflage applied at this early stage can also hide any bruising still evident, and thus prove a great morale booster.

Cosmetic camouflage differs considerably from ordinary cosmetic work. People asking for this service are distressed by some aspect of their appearance and the desired outcome of an interview with a cosmetician is that their confidence should be restored. They must therefore be considered as patients rather than as clients. These patients are inclined to be introverted, whereas clients seeking advice on make-up are of a more extrovert nature. Therefore with patients the cosmetician's approach has to be different, and she should correctly consider herself a clinical cosmetician with a particular role to play. She will need to become aware of the varying needs of her patients, which is less important where clients are concerned. Her patients will include men, women and children, all with one common factor – the need for help.

To see the patient's point of view, imagine what it must feel like to wake up after an accident to find one's own face or body mutilated. The initial shock to the system would inevitably be followed by natural reaction to that shock, producing mental anguish and possibly physical disorders as well.

There is a great human need to be acceptable in society, not only in appearance but also through personality, and there is no doubt that the two qualities are related. (Who has not felt better for being well dressed and well groomed and consequently more confident in company?) The human race has a peculiar tendency to judge its fellow beings by their appearance. So a particularly unfortunate situation must be where one of a pair of identical twins is born with an unsightly facial birthmark. The mental anguish suffered by the afflicted twin must be considerable, and the role of the parents in such a situation must also be particularly difficult.

The cosmetician's personality and her approach to patients play major roles in cosmetic camouflage therapy. The ability to look at appalling scars and also to touch them must be of paramount importance. Any tendency to flinch or show revulsion would be distressing to the patient, so the clinical cosmetician's reaction must always be positive and constructive, instilling confidence in the patient who, after all, comes in need of comfort and under-standing. The greatest triumphs from camouflage will come for those whose appearance may at first glance seem terrible. As is so often written in patients' notes, they need TLC – tender loving care!

Remedial camouflage is still considered by many people to be unnecessary and pandering to vanity. However, there are real and recognised symptoms of trauma and stress which can, indeed, be

present as a result of scarring. What may appear to be minor problems to some can mean much more to the afflicted.

This book sets out to give comprehensive instruction in the art of skin camouflage and will be useful to cosmeticians who wish to take up this specialism, either in hospitals or beauty salons. It also provides advice on techniques for individuals who are themselves scarred.

With so much movement of peoples between countries in the modern world, it is now extremely difficult to define particular skin colouring. Certainly the country of origin gives some indication of the depth of pigmentation present, but intermarriages, lifestyle, work and diet all play their part in producing different depths of colour in each individual's skin. I have therefore produced a chart with ten categories showing the range of possible colouring within countries given as examples.

Category A indicates the very palest possible skin shade, and Category J the darkest. Alongside the countries given as examples I have also listed the various shades of cover cream from which a skin colour match might be made.

For ease of reference this chart appears on p. 104, as well as on the accompanying bookmark.

2

The role of the clinical cosmetician

Why should this particular type of work be different from any other service provided by a cosmetician or beautician within a beauty establishment? A good working knowledge of cosmetics and their relative beneficial values or attributes is essential for any treatment and certainly a courteous approach should always be made to clients, whichever service they require.

Not all clients at a beauty establishment can be termed beautiful but this does not stop them booking appointments and enjoying the facilities, given that they can afford the treatment. However, the person seeking help to disguise a disfigurement would probably make the initial approach after a great deal of hesitancy, perhaps being unsure that such a service is available and reluctant to enter an establishment where only aids to beauty are being displayed. This first barrier can be overcome by a camouflage service being advertised in the window of the salon. At least then the first step can be taken confidently, in the knowledge that an initial enquiry will not bring a negative response.

Privacy is very important. People who are scarred can feel 'different' and even unacceptable in society, and may wish to hide, at least until the camouflage has been completed.

Remember that the patient who comes for advice on camouflage may differ considerably from the regular client attending for massage, sunbed and other treatments. Scarring affects people in all walks of life, and until a skin camouflage service is widely available everywhere, some patients will need to travel quite long distances in order to obtain help. Cost is therefore all-important – particularly to those who are managing on a limited budget. Not all camouflage patients fall into this category but it is advisable to assume at the beginning of the session that this may be the case. I would hope that any person giving a camouflage service would not wish to exclude a patient in need of help, simply because of a lack of financial resources. Scarring can so influence a patient's

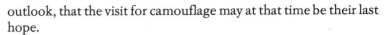

outlook, that the visit for camouflage may at that time be their last hope.

When you are working on camouflage for a patient, you will be thoroughly familiar with the routine but as, almost certainly, the patient will not, you will need to give detailed explanations of the procedure. Therefore you will need to assess how much information it will be possible for each patient to assimilate in each visit. Ultimately you will find that keeping the treatment as simple as possible will make it easier for the patient to copy.

From the cosmetician's point of view, the time allocated for a consultation must be carefully considered, allowing for the fact that, as in all businesses, time means money and affects profit. Nevertheless, I believe that cosmetic camouflage should be viewed more as a service than as a business proposition. The number of consultations for camouflage will be very small compared with those for other types of treatment but, in some cases, can produce further business from a satisfied client. Whenever possible, I would advise setting aside one hour for each patient, thus allowing ample time for assessing the patient's needs and yet ensuring the cosmetician time for trial and error in her treatment.

To summarise, each treatment needs to be unhurried, simple and reasonable. This policy should bring successful results – the patient having gained confidence and the cosmetician deep satisfaction.

APPROACH TO THE PATIENT

Your first priority in any interview should be to establish a rapport with the patient. This means particularly that you must project a positive attitude designed to instill confidence in your ability and willingness to help, remembering, nevertheless, that it is important not to make elaborate claims about the amount of success that can be assured. If promises of perfection are made, and then the results prove to be less than perfect, the effect on the patient could be catastrophic, particularly if the treatment was the patient's last hope. On the other hand, when a good working relationship has been established, the patient should have become involved in his or her own recovery or rehabilitation. By the end of the treatment, your patients must be able to carry out the camouflage themselves. They will then either be ready, with a more positive attitude, to start on the road to renewed confidence, or will at least have experienced a confidence not enjoyed before.

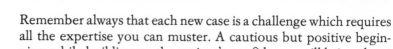

Remember always that each new case is a challenge which requires all the expertise you can muster. A cautious but positive beginning, while building up the patient's confidence, will bring about the best result.

Information regarding the scar to be treated may have been given at the time the appointment was made or in an accompanying letter from a doctor. If this has not been done and the area of scarring is still unknown, it is essential to leave the patients to explain their own requirements. The particular problem concerning them may not be immediately apparent and, indeed, an apparent defect that is obvious to the cosmetician may not prove to be the problem worrying the patient. Not only can a wrong assessment be made inopportunely, causing both patient and cosmetician embarrassment, but some harm might be done by attention being called to a secondary defect.

GREATER AWARENESS

Once you have embarked on cosmetic camouflage therapy as a career, you will develop a greater awareness of physical defects in others. When you meet strangers with scarring your natural reaction may be to offer unsolicited help. But first consider carefully the person who has learned either to live with scarring or even to be no longer aware of something which may cause revulsion in others. Drawing attention to the defect can cause immeasurable harm, even though this is done from an honest desire to help. So remember that just as you should leave patients to explain their own requirements from camouflage, you should give the same consideration to casual acquaintances or strangers.

CONTACT WITH GPs

Patients may present themselves for treatment without having first consulted a doctor; it may be that their scarring was sustained a number of years previously, or was congenital, or even that they are too embarrassed to approach more than one person about it. Indeed, many doctors are unaware that positive help is available and will merely advise patients that nothing can be done and that they 'must learn to live with it'. This situation should occur less as cosmetic camouflage becomes better understood and is accepted as a natural right for all patients. The greater the number of patients who do receive these treatments and the more who know

about them, the better. This will help to improve the present situation and dispel ignorance on the subject. Cosmeticians can themselves play a part in spreading the knowledge of such a service by always informing the GP concerned of the treatment given to his or her patient. However, this should not be the prime reason for keeping the doctor informed. It may be that medical treatment and cosmetic camouflage will together bring about an even better end result, so a referral to the doctor should be carried out as a matter of principle for all patients.

The question of safety of both patient and cosmetician is all-important. Should a cosmetician not involve the medical practitioner in the treatment, both she and the patient could be affected by the consequences of negligence. The following case underlines this point. Sensitivity to sunlight can produce the common skin condition known as vitiligo, which results in pure white areas appearing on the skin, particularly on the face and hands. Vitiligo is not infectious or contagious, and gives the patient no physical discomfort. At present there is no cure for it. The point to note, however, is that at its onset one form of leprosy has exactly the same appearance as vitiligo. The only difference is that with leprosy there is a loss of sensation in the affected areas. While leprosy is very uncommon in developed countries, this case illustrates the point that without medical knowledge the cosmetician cannot be too careful. If the patient had seen a doctor, the complaint would have been correctly diagnosed – certainly no case of leprosy would be referred for camouflage.

The conclusion must be that all patients should be seen on doctors' referrals and, where none has been made, contact should be made with the GP before treatment is given.

UNDERLYING PROBLEMS

Familiarity with camouflage therapy will bring with it an appreciation of any possible underlying problems. In many cases these problems may prove to be psychological, perhaps springing from the erroneous belief that failure to achieve a personal ambition is due to some adverse aspect of the appearance. Hopefully, the cosmetician will be able to overcome this by her contribution to an improved appearance. However, medical knowledge might be required to find out the underlying cause of the problem, so it is essential that the principle of referral be adhered to at all times. This will happen as a matter of course when the cosmetician is working within a hospital or medical practice, where qualified guidance will always be at hand.

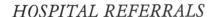

HOSPITAL REFERRALS

In a hospital situation referrals will be made by either the consultant dermatologist or the consultant plastic surgeon. The camouflage clinic is usually run alongside one of these consultants' outpatient clinics, which are normally held once a week. Early on in her career, attendance by the cosmetician will probably be necessary only once a month. As she gains experience, so the cosmetician may be requested to make more frequent attendances, with an increasing number of referrals being made to her, with her workload expanding to include patients from other clinics such as endocrinology, general surgery and paediatrics. The cosmetician may also be asked to visit in-patients undergoing treatment on the wards, in order to tell them about the possibility of camouflage at a later stage of their rehabilitation. This can be a great morale booster for the patients when their need for reassurance is utmost.

TYPES OF PATIENT

Men

It is a fact that as many men will seek assistance as do women and children, which is not so surprising when one considers that the majority of drivers are men and it is predominantly men who will be injured in warfare, flying and mining accidents as well as in disasters at sea. Because appearances can so affect job opportunities, men are now more conscious of the image they project. Obviously basic and undetectable camouflage is what is required for their treatment. Sometimes the male approach can be rather tentative and reassurance should be given that the number of male patients certainly equals that of females, and that the service offered is different from make-up.

Women

Female patients are usually less inhibited than males about seeing the cosmetician and, after the camouflage is completed satisfactorily, will often ask advice on make-up and general skin problems. Women through the ages have accepted the use of cosmetics and are usually anxious to receive any tips on the possible improvement of any aspect of their appearance, including hair-style and care, colour of clothing and so on. Nevertheless it can be prudent to hold back suggestions unless advice is invited by the patient, who might otherwise feel that unsolicited advice was unwanted criticism.

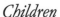
Showing a child how to camouflage a defect can bring enormous benefit, but if he or she is made to feel 'different' or inferior because of the camouflage, the treatment could have the opposite effect, possibly causing an inferiority complex for life. No child should ever be made to feel unacceptable without camouflage.

In the case of a child with a birthmark, the parents may have suffered feelings of shame or guilt which have prompted them to seek the help of camouflage. It is important that they should be made aware of all that can be done to hide the offending mark, but if the child is still too young to apply the cream for him or herself, you can suggest that a return visit at a later date might prove more helpful. The reasons should be explained fully to the parents, and you can suggest that they return either when the child is due to start school or if the child expresses a desire to hide the mark.

Many birthmarks will disappear quite naturally within the first few years of life and because of this, many people will not be aware that such a mark ever existed. Thought should therefore be given to camouflage being applied to younger children when, on special occasions, photographs might be taken. If camouflage has been applied before photographs are taken in childhood, no historical evidence of the birthmark will remain, which is particularly important where the mark disappears naturally during childhood. Indeed, even if the mark does not disappear but is being cleverly camouflaged, no one other than the patient need be aware that it has ever existed. Children who prefer not to bother with cover creams in their early years may change their views as they grow up. Their attitude toward their scarring may be affected by chance unkind remarks from others, or in teenage years when they become more aware of their appearance. At this stage you might consider devising a programme using very little cover initially and increasing it little by little over several weeks, so that the mark disappears very gradually. It is always worthwhile suggesting this slow method as an alternative to immediate and complete cover, because it should cause less embarassment and might go unnoticed, with the original mark being forgotten by others during the process of gradual disguise.

RECORDS

Care must be taken in the detailed recording of the extent of the scarring of each patient, together with the treatment which is

given and how successful the result proves to be. Equally important is the need to make sure the patient is fully aware of the complete procedure. Written details of the procedure should be supplied at the end of the session, together with details of the creams that were chosen and where further supplies can be obtained. Sample cards for these two purposes are shown below and opposite.

YOUR REFERENCE CARD

Patient's name

Address and tel. no.

Age

Source of referral

Name of doctor

Doctor's address and tel. no.

Extent of scarring

Creams used

Number of applications

Method

Result

Information sent

Fee charged   Date

The reverse side should list the date(s) and time(s) of appointments.

A detailed report of the treatment given and the result obtained should be sent to the patient's doctor so that he or she will know whether any follow up or further medical treatment is required, and whether camouflage has proved completely satisfactory to the

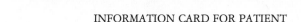

INFORMATION CARD FOR PATIENT

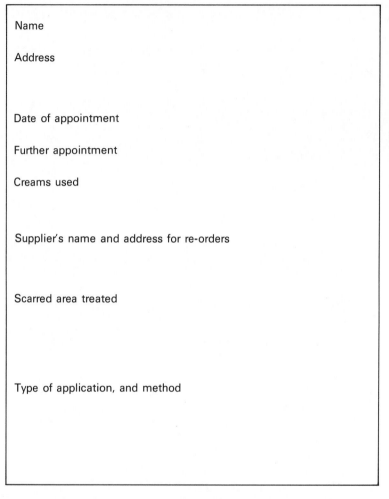

Name

Address

Date of appointment

Further appointment

Creams used

Supplier's name and address for re-orders

Scarred area treated

Type of application, and method

patient. If creams are to be obtained by prescription from the doctor, as is the case in the United Kingdom where the costs are covered by the National Health Service, then full details will be needed in the report.

Where the supplies of creams are held in stock by the cosmetician, a stock sheet should be kept with details of all the stock held and a note made of when re-ordering will be necessary and also when orders are made and received.

3

Your basic kit

This chapter deals with the equipment that you will need to give a full cosmetic camouflage service to the patient. To achieve a really good result you will also require an inventive approach, but a basic set of equipment must always be available to meet every possible requirement.

The container for the equipment and preparations will, naturally, be a matter of choice. If you are to work in a salon or a place in which your materials can always be at hand, then a dental trolley or similar unit is ideal, provided that it has sufficiently deep drawers for displaying all the creams, etc., that you will need, both for your own convenience and that of your patient.

Often, however, it is more convenient to have a portable unit. This will need to be roomy and lightweight but robust. Beauty boxes are generally too small and they lack the necessary display compartments to enable you to have the range of creams, etc., ready to hand. An ideal solution can be found in the most unlikely places: a lightweight plastic case of the type used by electricians is widely available at builders merchants and hardware stores and serves the purpose admirably. It is compact when closed, being only about 15 cm wide by 50 cm long, but opens to reveal three removable trays: one deep and two shallow, with the base as a further compartment. The case is relatively strong, easily cleaned and, being made of plastic, adds little to the considerable weight of the equipment to be transported.

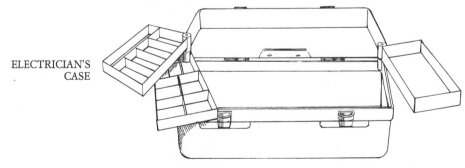

ELECTRICIAN'S
CASE

Alternatively you may wish to consider plastic fishing tackle boxes, which are available in the United Kingdom in two sizes and obtainable in many stores.

Whatever you choose, remember that there may be times when no facilities will be available when you attend a patient and therefore the portable container should be big enough to accommodate at least a little of everything that might be required. Time taken in choosing a satisfactory case will not be wasted. Perhaps the most sensible approach would first be to collect together all the items that have to fit into the case, thus giving you a clearer idea of exactly what is needed.

First and foremost you will need the samples of all the cover creams that you use. Some manufacturers have made the task easier by producing small and easily transportable sample kits, which can be easily refilled as necessary from a larger stock kept at home. (You may also decide to hold your own bulk stock of the various creams, so that a patient can purchase these from you for immediate use. To keep the whole range might prove prohibitively expensive, but there are some shades that are used more frequently than others.)

You will need to carry with you information to give to patients on where they can obtain the various creams you find suitable for them. In most cases, because of their limited market, these will not be available from retailers, since most retailers favour commodities that will sell quickly rather than holding stocks with limited appeal. In some hospitals you may be able to arrange for the pharmacist to carry a stock of creams to provide patients with an initial supply. Thereafter they will need to obtain their creams either on prescription from their GP, as in the United Kingdom under the National Health Service, or by private purchase.

In view of the relative difficulty of obtaining the creams, you may consider it worthwhile to carry a small empty container in your kit. You can then supply a patient with a small quantity of cream from your own kit, to give them the confidence to attend a special function, for example, before they are able to obtain their own supply.

You will need a pot of removal cream, or any bland cleansing cream, to remove all traces of dirt and prepare the skin before you apply camouflage. Also have a bottle each of witch hazel and rose water for removing oil from the skin, otherwise the camouflage creams could 'slide' on application and be unstable.

You will find it convenient to have a supply of damp cotton wool swabs prepared in advance of your appointments. These are made

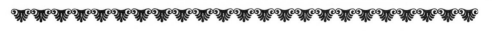

by cutting a large roll of cotton wool (a) into approximately 10 cm strips crosswise (b), and in turn cutting these into three (c) and making swabs of approximately 10 cm square (d). Soak swabs in water, then squeeze as dry as possible (e), so that when stored in a suitable container, they can be peeled off in thin layers as required.

A plastic box approximately 10 cm square by 5 cm deep is an ideal container, which will hold as many prepared swabs as you are likely to need for up to five or six patients.

It may be necessary to camouflage a mark in an area where other natural and acceptable blemishes – such as freckles and so on – will continue to exist alongside the camouflage. In these cases the now faultless camouflage must not only hide the mark but must also be made to match the surrounding imperfections. This is called 'faking faults'. Several natural cosmetic sponges kept in a plastic bag are particularly useful when faking these faults and sometimes for applying the basic cover cream when only a light covering is necessary. It is advisable to wash these sponges as soon as possible after use, using toilet soap and warm water to ease out the colouring matter. After cleansing, the sponges should be placed in mild antiseptic solution for a minimum of 10 minutes before further use.

You will need at least twelve small brushes for application of the cover creams. Lip brushes are ideal, particularly those that are wide but flat. An alternative would be artists' brushes. In the United Kingdom, Windsor & Newton produce a shaped brush called Series 52 of which sizes four, five and six prove the most useful. A shaped brush is necessary when applying cream to thin hairline-type scars, as well as for patch colour testing. All brushes should be cleansed and sterilised in the same manner as cosmetic sponges. You will therefore need with you a tablet of toilet soap in a container and a supply of mild antiseptic. You may also feel it is prudent to carry a small quantity of water in case you find yourself short of basic facilities at the time of the consultation.

For fixing or setting the cover creams after application some powder is essential. Non-perfumed talcum powder is one possibility, and a little can be transferred to a small plastic container if space is limited. Occasionally you may find that a better result can be obtained with translucent powder, particularly on a black skin. Some manufacturers of cover creams supply a special finishing powder. Less expensive than this and obtainable in the United Kingdom is Theatrical Blending Powder No. 1183 Neutral, produced by Innoxa under their Leichner label and marketed in 200 g packs. Other alternatives are Kryolan translucent (from West

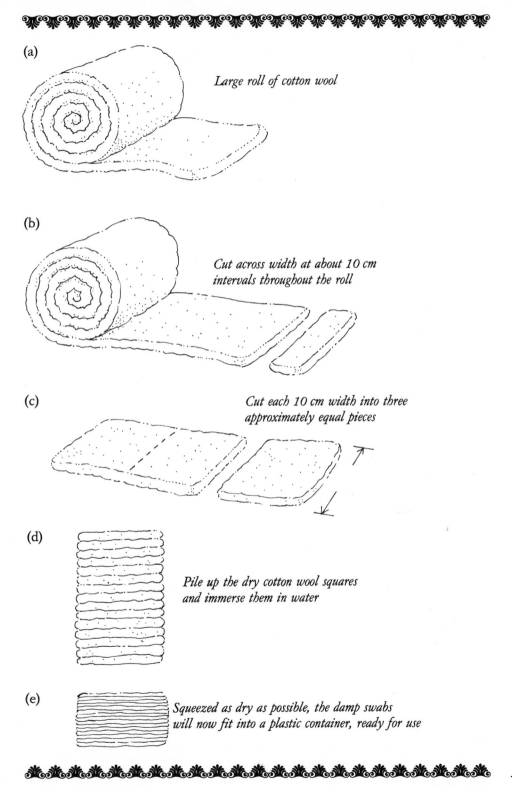

(a) Large roll of cotton wool

(b) Cut across width at about 10 cm intervals throughout the roll

(c) Cut each 10 cm width into three approximately equal pieces

(d) Pile up the dry cotton wool squares and immerse them in water

(e) Squeezed as dry as possible, the damp swabs will now fit into a plastic container, ready for use

Germany) or Max Factor translucent Beige (United Kingdom and United States). In the United Kingdom all these powders are available from Charles Fox Ltd, 22 Tavistock Street, London, WC2E 7PY (telephone 01-240 3111) as well as through some of the larger chemists and department stores. Any one of these products will suit your needs. For applying them you will need a supply of dry cotton wool.

There is no need to carry a wide range of cosmetics since you will find these are rarely needed. The following basic pack should be sufficient: a choice of two lipsticks, one pale, one bright, together with a lip pencil; black block mascara with a small separate brush which can be washed and sterilised after use and a small container of water for its application; one block of powder blusher; powder block eyeshadow in, for example, grey-green, blue-grey and light brown.

When you come to faking faults after the cover cream has been applied, some cream-based rouge and a cream-based navy blue eyeshadow are useful. Occasionally a patient may suffer a loss of pigment to the eyelashes as a result of vitiligo and it can be helpful to have with you a supply of black eyelash dye, together with a small bottle of 20 vol. hydrogen peroxide.

You should always carry a basic supply of prosthetics: one set of false nails; a set of daytime eyelashes and fixative; a small amount each of the five available colours of crepe hair (such as that used in stage and TV make-up) together with a bottle of spirit gum for application. (Crepe hair and spirit gum are available in the United Kingdom from Charles Fox and in other countries from established theatrical make-up agents.)

A section of the case can be devoted to the small number of implements that you will require: a few orange sticks for extracting the cover creams; a wooden spatula for the cleansing cream; small sharp scissors for trimming false eyelashes, nails or crepe hair; and record cards for your notes. You will find the palm of your hand is adequate for mixing colours. Finally, and this is most important, you should carry a mirror so that patients can watch what you are doing when working on their faces.

Amazingly, all these items fit quite easily into one of the boxes already described. With this kit you will be able to travel with confidence to treat your patients, whether they are in a hospital or their own homes.

This is a summary of what you will need in your lightweight carrying box.

Samples of cover cream
Cleansing cream
Rose water
Witch hazel
Plastic box containing damp prepared cotton wool swabs
Natural cosmetic sponges – say four
12 lip brushes
Talcum powder (unscented if possible)
Translucent powder or finishing powder, now available from all
   manufacturers mentioned in this book
Dry cotton wool
Cream rouge (Dermacolor D32, Covermark rouge or Veil Rose)
Navy blue cream-based eyeshadow
2 lipsticks – 1 pale, 1 bright
1 lip pencil
Black block mascara
Powder block eyeshadow – say grey-green, blue-grey and light
   brown
Powder block blusher
Black eyelash dye – vegetable base
20 vol. peroxide (for use with dye)
1 set false nails
1 set daytime eyelashes and fixative
Crepe hair – 5 colours
Spirit gum
Water
Tablet toilet soap in plastic container
Antiseptic
Mirror
Orange sticks
Wooden spatula
Pair small sharp scissors
Writing pad
Record cards – yours and patients'
Pen
Small empty container to give cream sample to patient

4

Cover creams

In mentioning particular types of cover cream, inevitably some of those currently available in various parts of the world will be omitted. Most well-known manufacturers of ordinary cosmetics now produce cover creams which have the covering properties necessary for camouflage and it is the task of the cosmetician embarking on this work to find out about them and where samples are available. She must obtain the creams to assess their stability in wear and must also ascertain whether they are waterproof and sunproof. In other words as a cosmetician you should familiarise yourself with all available creams before choosing those you will work with. Manufacturers are always prepared to explain their products and supply written information about them.

After obtaining several brands of cream you can compare the differences in texture between them. The ointment base differs noticeably between products, and while some will flow on easily, others will appear 'tacky' and be less easy to spread, making the covering of a large area of scarring quite difficult.

However, despite differences in their consistency, camouflage creams usually have two common factors. Firstly, the majority are waterproofed to enable the wearer to participate in all manner of activities, including swimming and water sports, with complete confidence in the stability of the product. Secondly, the creams are sunproofed, most of them containing titanium dioxide as an ultra-violet reflectant to protect scar tissue from the harmful ultra-violet rays of sunlight. Over-exposure to sunlight is dangerous for normal skin, not only because its drying effect causes premature ageing but because of the possible effect of radiation which can cause changes to occur in the structure of the skin. Where scar tissue is present it is necessary to take particular care. It is easy to see what a difference use of these creams can make to the lifestyle of the wearer.

Camouflage on the face must be applied daily and, ideally, removed at night – natural perspiration together with dirt would

clog the pores of the skin and might lead to further problems. However, some patients, particularly those with large amounts of scarring, elect to use their camouflage at all times, reapplying it immediately after removal and cleansing. Used in this way cover creams cause no harm to the skin.

On the other hand, where camouflage creams are used on other parts of the body, they will sometimes give excellent coverage over a number of days without removal – as long as the wearer is careful not to use soap on the treated areas when washing, showering or bathing. Because soap tends to dislodge the creams – although it will not remove them completely – it will spoil the cover by disturbing some of the cream and producing a patchy effect. When drying with a towel after bathing, a blotting – rather than a rubbing – action should be used.

It must be noted that a patient with a drier type of skin will find the cover creams more efficient over a longer period than those patients who have an oily type of skin. The increased production of sebum in patients with oily skins tends to lift the cover in a shorter time by mixing with the cream and 'thinning' it. Cover creams are removed by the application of a cream cleanser, the active ingredient being the oil they contain, so where the skin is naturally oily, cover creams can tend to be less stable and patients should be told of this probability and the possible need for more frequent applications to maintain a good cover.

Climate too has to be considered. This can have an effect on the stability of the creams. Those who live in a cold climate will find the camouflage more effective over a longer period than those who live in a hot climate where perspiration, because of its oily consistency, will inevitably loosen the creams more quickly. While cover creams contain no healing properties, they do not harm the skin and although water cannot penetrate them, the normal function of perspiration can continue unhindered. Patients should always be made aware of all the points relevant to their particular lifestyle.

With the many ranges of cover cream now available, there is an ever increasing choice of colours from which to select, making it easier for the cosmetician to match exactly the patient's own skin tone in the area surrounding the scar tissue. Where there is no exact matching shade available, you will need to mix colours together in varying quantities. In the case of the required shade falling, say, half way between two available shades, a mix of equal parts of both may prove to be exactly right. Ideally, the colour you choose or mix should blend in with the surrounding tissue and be

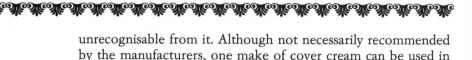

unrecognisable from it. Although not necessarily recommended by the manufacturers, one make of cover cream can be used in conjunction with others, with excellent results.

To assist you in the selection of creams, below are listed the most significant products, with as much detail as possible of their availability and range. When you become familiar with the various creams, you will be able to decide which ones to include in your working kit and which ones to discard.

VEIL COVER CREAM (SCALE A–H)

Veil Cover Cream is produced by Thomas Blake & Co., Blatchford Close, Horsham, Sussex, RH13 5RQ, England (tel. Horsham (0403) 54742). An excellent cream with a fine ointment base, it is produced in ten basic skin tones. Originally marketed in seven skin shades and pure white, the range now includes extra colours – brown, olive green, yellow and rose – making it suitable for a wide range of skin colouring.

The basic colours are called Medium, Tan, Dark, Suntan, Natural, Natural-Medium, Natural-Tan and White. The two deeper colours are called simply Dark Numbers 2 and 3. (See colour chart, p. 104, for suitability.)

Complete sample kits are supplied free of charge to hospitals and clinics and are available to the general public at a very reasonable cost (currently £4.00). For beauticians a sample kit will be supplied free of charge with any initial order of twenty-four jars, whereas a small sample of each colour will be supplied to anyone sending a S.A.E. and enclosing 50p towards the cost of the samples.

This cream is most suitable for small blemishes or where only a very light cover is required – such as for the condition known as rosacea, where the whole area of the face is affected and needs only 'toning down' – rather than a solid cover that would give a mask-like effect. Veil is both waterproof and resistant to ultra-violet light. It is available by post from the manufacturers within a matter of days and is available in the United Kingdom on prescription under the National Health Service. The smallest, 19 g, size retails currently at £2.00, including postage, packing and VAT. The largest, 70 g, size is currently £4.00, making this product the cheapest one available. It is also obtainable in a limited number of retail outlets in the United Kingdom, including some chemists and

salons. This company now produces a cleansing cream, which is unperfumed and is a water-in-oil product. It retails currently at £2.50 for a 100 g jar. Thomas Blake, the manufacturers of Veil Cover Cream, have added a translucent finishing powder and a toning lotion to their range.

COVERMARK COVER CREAM (SCALE A–I)

Covermark Cover Cream is licensed by Lydia O'Leary of 41 East 57th Street, New York, NY10022, USA. The sole distributors in the United Kingdom are Medexport Ltd, PO Box 25, Arundel, West Sussex, BN18 0SW, England, for orders both in the United Kingdom and overseas (for countries other than those listed below). For limited purchases this cream is obtainable in London for personal shoppers – cash sales only – from Medexport Ltd, at 76 Wells Street, London W1P 3RE, (tel. 01–637 3169 and 01–580 6375).

In Canada enquiries should be made to Professional Pharmacy Corporation, 2795 Bates Road, Montreal 26.

In Hawaii enquiries should be made to Lydia O'Leary, 1234 Ala Moana Center, 1450 Ala Moana Boulevard, Honolulu 96814, (tel. 993288).

In Japan enquiries should be made to Pias Corporation, 21–3, 3 Chome, Toyasaki, Oyodu-Ku, Osaka.

In Iran enquiries should be made to Alosen Co., 58 Madaen St, Jam Avenue, Takhte-Tavoos, Teheran 15.

Covermark has a fairly thick ointment base with good covering qualities. It is produced in nine basic shades in 25 g pots only, from very pale through to very dark colours, and also in pure white. Also available are three rouges: blonde, medium and brunette; a grey toner for stimulating 'five o'clock shadows' on men, and a shading cream most useful for the simulation of natural shadows around eyes, nose and chin to obtain a natural finish on the face.

The skin shades are called Light, Peach, Medium, Brunette, Rose-Dark, Dark Brown, Number 1, Number 8 and Number 3 (a very dark brown colour). This company also produces its own finishing powder and removal cream. All the products including the cover creams are formulated to be non-allergenic and non-irritant. Covermark Cover Cream is also waterproof and resistant to sunlight and abrasion.

Covermark is also produced in a stick form called Spotstik, which is useful for small blemishes, dark circles round the eyes, bruises, pimples and suchlike. Spotstik comes in seven shades including Light, Medium, Brunette, Dark, Suntan, Number 8 and Bronze.

The basic masking creams are more expensive than the rouges and toners, but as this product is listed in MIMS (*Monthly Index of Medical Specialities*), the manual of prescribable products for UK doctors, it is obtainable on prescription through the National Health Service.

Covermark is probably the most widely known product for cosmetic camouflage and is particularly useful for camouflage on skins scale F–J, having four excellent colours for this purpose (Dark Brown, Numbers 1, 8 and 3).

This cream can be obtained from the distributors in a demonstration kit, which includes all the available shades of cover cream, toners and rouges as well as setting powder. There is a reduction in the price of these demonstration kits when a large number is ordered for a school or training establishment. Colour cards showing the full Covermark range are also available on request from the distributors together with the current price list.

Medexport Ltd sponsor Covermark Certificate Courses, and from students who have attended the course have compiled a register of trained personnel in the United Kingdom available for patients seeking help within the private sector.

Courses are available on a regular basis at the Covermark Training School (a Division of DuBarry International Ltd), Arundel College, River Road Campus, Arundel, W. Sussex BN18 9EY. Courses are also run at intervals in Birmingham, Manchester, Cardiff and Glasgow and can be made available by arrangement at other centres in the United Kingdom. One-day Covermark orientation courses are provided for medical personnel as well as certificated courses for those with acceptable previous experience. Enquiries regarding courses should be made to The Director of Training, Medexport Ltd, PO Box 25, Arundel, W. Sussex BN18 0SW.

KEROMASK COVER CREAM (SCALE A–J)

Keromask Cover Cream is produced by Innoxa (England) Ltd, 202 Terminus Road, Eastbourne, Sussex BN21 3DF, England (tel. 0323 639671, international telegrams: Interbeauty Eastbourne, Telex 87682). All orders and enquiries both from the United

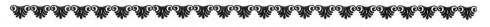

Kingdom and abroad should be made to this address initially, although Keromask is available in many overseas countries, where an exclusive arrangement has been made with a local organisation (for example, Belgium, the Netherlands, Nigeria, Oman, Malaysia, Hong Kong and Singapore). All enquiries regarding specific countries should be made to the Group Overseas Marketing Manager, Innoxa (England) Ltd (address on p. 22).

Keromask has a fairly thick ointment base (although slightly thinner than Covermark) and is easily spread, giving excellent coverage particularly of port-wine stains and naevi. It is also recommended for disorders of pigmentation such as vitiligo, leucoderma, broken veins and abnormally coloured skin often associated with pregnancy. The ochre pigments used in this product are of the iron-oxide type in order to reduce to a minimum the possibility of any sensitisation reaction. This cream is both waterproof and resistant to sunlight. Keromask is produced in eight colours, three of them being used as masking creams to obliterate blemishes and five being toning products to adjust the colour of the masked area to the surrounding skin. Three premix colours – light, medium and dark – have now been added to the range. It is suggested that these can be used to cover small blemishes in the most nearly matching skin tone. They can also be premixed with other colours in the range to effect a perfect skin match for larger areas. Innoxa suggest that each individual normally requires four colours, depending on the part of the face or body to be covered, as well as on the skin colouring of the patient. The colours available are Brown (No. 1), White (No. 2), Honey (No. 3), Rose (No. 4), Yellow (No. 5), Black (No. 6), Chestnut (No. 7) and Umber (No. 8). The new premix shades are Light (No. 9), Medium (No. 10) and Dark (No. 11). For skins in the scale A–F inclusive, first use either Brown (No. 1) or White (No. 2) to mask the scarred area, whereas for skins in categories G–J first use Chestnut (No. 7). A small quantity of the base is rubbed well in until the mark is completely obliterated. Toning colours are then applied over the base colour in order to match the surrounding skin area. Honey and Rose are generally suggested for facial blemishes, with Yellow used for the body and for all areas of skins in categories E–H. Black is used for shading areas such as the beard line on men, whereas Umber is used in conjunction with Chestnut on skins in categories H–J.

Innoxa suggest that there is no need to use a setting powder with camouflage on male patients, although where the affected areas are in contact with clothing, powdering and setting the cream would seem to be necessary to protect clothing which might otherwise become soiled. Constant contact with clothing also tends to erase the cover cream if setting with powder has not been carried out. A new finishing powder has therefore been introduced for setting the creams.

Although Keromask is claimed by the manufacturer to be stable for one day only, it has proved to last for a number of days without renewal on such areas as the hands and legs – even with daily bathing.

No sample kits of Keromask are produced, although from time to time demonstrations are arranged for the product, and the company has compiled a list of cosmeticians who have attended such demonstrations and to whom the public can be referred.

Keromask is listed in MIMS and is therefore obtainable in the United Kingdom on prescription from a doctor. In the United Kingdom this product is sometimes held in small quantities in department stores or by chemists who have an Innoxa cosmetic stand.

DERMACOLOR COVER CREAM (SCALE A–J)

Dermacolor Cover Cream is produced by Kryolan GmbH, Papierstrasse 10, D1000, Berlin 51, West Germany, a company famous for its stage and theatrical products. In the United Kingdom the sole distributors are Charles Fox Ltd, 22 Tavistock Street, London WC2.

This cream is also available in the following countries:

Australia Dermacolor Camouflage System, Marylin Cunnington, 45 Repton Road, East Malvern Victoria 3145

United States Kryolan Corporation, 747 Polk Street, San Francisco, California 94109

South Africa Kryolan (SA) PTY Ltd, Siegi's Make-up Centre, 45 Kruis St, Johannesburg, TVL 2001

Finland Firma, Koukkanen Peruukkiliike Ky., It. Teatterikiya 5B, Helsinki 10

Canada Malabar Ltd, 14 McCaul Street, Toronto 28, Ontario

Argentina Sra Elena Wegelin de Gori, Buenos Aires 3180 RA – 1636 Olivos

Norway Firma., A/S Frisor, Youngsgatan 11B., N-Oslo 1

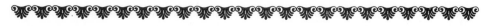

Netherlands Firma., Impex, B.Knispel-Couperus, Bernisse 1, Zwolle, Nederland

Dermacolor can also be obtained in Austria, Belgium, Switzerland and the Republic of Ireland through main Kryolan make-up agents.

This cream has a fine ointment base with excellent covering qualities and is produced in a comprehensive range of colours totalling twenty-six basic skin shades, ranging from very pale to very dark. Also offered in the range are seven toners including off-white (D0) and black (D40) together with several colours for shading. Particularly useful as a first coat over the red dye of tattoos is an eau-de-nil shade called 1742. A new addition called 406 is a porcelain colour for use on shiny skin (burns), before covering with a matching skin colour.

Kryolan produces a variety of sample kits, starting with a handy pocket-size plastic container holding sixteen colours from the range. Larger metal sample boxes are also available in several sizes with varying numbers of the creams included in larger quantities.

This cream is sold in 1 oz jars and is in the medium to high price range, although in the United Kingdom it is available on prescription through the National Health Service, as is their setting powder. It has the advantage of being suitable for most types of scarring, and its availability in so many countries as well as its wide range of colours make it an excellent product. This cover cream is both waterproof and resistant to sunlight. It is applied in the usual manner and is 'set' for stability in the normal way.

As well as their large range of cover creams, Kryolan also include fixing powder, cleansing cream and cleansing milk for use with their cream as well as skin plastic in three shades for filling holes. Skin plastic has proved to be unsuitable for masking acne pitting, in that it stays soft and marks on touch. Although make-up can be applied over skin plastic, it would probably have only limited use, except on very deep scarring – where plastic surgery would seem to be a better and permanent solution. For extra stability in hot climates and to reduce the effects of perspiration on the camouflage, a Fixier spray has been produced.

DERMABLEND COVER CREAM (SCALE C–I)

Dermablend Cover Cream is a recent addition to the range of camouflage creams, manufactured by the Flori Roberts Co., Box 758, Farmingdale, New Jersey, USA 07727. It has recently become available in the United Kingdom and enquiries should be made to Flori Roberts, Director of Corrective Cosmetics, 31 Charles Street, Mayfair, London W1X 7PN (tel. 01-493 7942/3).

The company is well known for its range of cosmetics designed for skins in categories F–J, and other beauty preparations including Chromatone Plus which, it is claimed, will fade hyperpigmentation in skins affected by freckles, age spots and uneven skin tone. Dermablend is produced in eight shades named Chroma 1 to Chroma 7. Chroma 1, 2, 2A and 3 could be used to match skins in categories C–G, with Chroma 4 to Chroma 7 being used for more deeply pigmented skins, categories G–I. This cream is not available on prescription in the United Kingdom. It is supplied in 1½ oz jars for private purchase and is in the higher price range. Small trial (¼ oz) are available in all eight shades.

Dermablend is waterproof and non-greasy, resistant to sunlight and smudging and will not rub off on clothing. It is also free of fragrance. The Flori Roberts range for camouflage includes a setting powder and a cream remover called Melanin Cleanser.

If ordinary make-up is to be used over this cover cream, a hydrophilic foundation is recommended and this is also produced by the same manufacturers.

BOOTS COVER CREAM (SCALE C–E)

In the United Kingdom, Boots the Chemists produce a small range of four colours of cover cream. However, although this product is readily obtainable over the counter, it tends to be rather thick and is not claimed to be waterproof.

5

Mixing and matching the creams

Expertise in camouflage therapy comes from repeated practice but one important attribute for the cosmetician is an awareness of colour. It will take time for you to recognise the various shades which each contribute to a particular skin tone. Also the shade which might seem correct before application to the skin can appear entirely different when it is actually applied to the scarred area.

Most probably you will have had the experience, for instance when buying a lipstick, of choosing a shade which is pale pink in the container, but proves to be a more harsh and brighter colour when applied to your lips. This effect is caused by the amount of acid present in your skin, so that the same shade of lipstick will appear quite different on different people. Cover creams can also undergo a colour change. After applying a cream to a small test patch adjacent to a scar, wait a few minutes before you judge the suitability of the shade. Sometimes the creams may appear to turn rather pink or even grey. It is wise to try cream from an alternative range at this point to see if that too behaves in the same way.

One easy way to learn about colour is to experiment with a child's set of coloured paints, and become familiar with the results of mixing colours together. After repeated trials you will see what results can be expected.

The best way to approach this subject is to use only the primary colours, of which there are three – red, yellow and blue. From these colours, you will rediscover the excitement of mixing to produce completely new shades. Water-colour paints are ideal, being very simple to mix for the following experiments.

Start by mixing together the blue and yellow, in equal proportions; the result will be a mid-green. When you mix blue and red in the same way you will have a rich purple; equal proportions of red and yellow mixed together give a rich orange.

Now take this a step further and discover how, still by mixing only

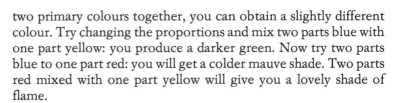

two primary colours together, you can obtain a slightly different colour. Try changing the proportions and mix two parts blue with one part yellow: you produce a darker green. Now try two parts blue to one part red: you will get a colder mauve shade. Two parts red mixed with one part yellow will give you a lovely shade of flame.

Continue experimenting with just these three primary colours, using them in pairs in varying proportions together. Literally hundreds of different shades can be produced and if you note carefully the basic mix you use, you can repeat these shades accurately over and over again.

During this first set of experiments you have used only two colours mixed together, but now consider adding to these a proportion of pure white. Start again with equal proportions of two of the primary colours, and add an equal amount of white to each mix. See how once again you have produced a new colour, which is more delicate than before. Continue through the various mixes you used previously, but each time add an equal amount of white. Try varying the proportions and note carefully how each new shade was achieved.

Gradually you will develop a new feeling for colour, and by covering up the details of how each shade was produced, you can test yourself to see if you can recognise the colours and proportions you have used in each case. When you have reached the stage where you can confidently recognise the mixes you used and their proportions, it will be time to move on to the next step.

The reason behind these tests may still appear to be rather obscure and to bear no relation to the business of matching skin tones and cover creams. However, if you take the time and trouble to try these basic mixes, the reason for the tests will become apparent.

So far only two primary colours have been used together in one mix, with the addition of white. Now continue with the next step, mixing the three primary colours together in equal proportions. The result will be a muddy dark brown colour, which resembles a very dark skin colour.

Now use the three primary colours together but vary the proportions. Start by using twice as much yellow as the other two colours. Follow this by making a mix of two parts blue to one each of red and yellow, and lastly try a mix with two parts red to one each of blue and yellow. As with the previous set of mixes, you can try adding a single part of white to each of these combinations. By altering all the various proportions you will see that the possibilities are

endless, and that the more tests you do, the more you will learn about how the various manufacturers produce their ranges of skin colours. You will also see how easy it is to change slightly a given colour so that it will exactly match a patient's skin. Familiarity and practice will make it easier for you to see which colour needs to be added.

Therefore, when no exact colour match is available in any particular type of cream, the addition of a small amount of one of the primary colours can give you an exact match. For instance the Keromask Cover Cream range includes Yellow (No. 5), Rose (No. 4) (a vivid red) and Chestnut (No. 7) (a mixture of both red and yellow). Together with pure white – produced by most manufacturers – these creams will allow almost any skin colour to be produced accurately. Even though no manufacturers presently provide a blue cover cream, nevertheless blue is in some basic shades and these can be used in a mix as necessary. If you spend time playing with colour in this way, you will learn a tremendous amount. It is worth remembering that the things we do not know or understand may seem impossible but become second nature as we really understand them. The desire to understand expresses all the so-called 'talent' one needs – but without practice, the desire is useless.

Having understood how cover creams are produced in various depths of colour, thought must be given to the colouring you will find in the skin of your patients.

SKINS SCALE A–D

In skins with this range (see colour chart, p. 104) it is easy to see the various shades which are present. Firstly there is blue and pink from the blood capillaries, which show up almost in a pattern or network. Behind this will be the basic tone, generally of a very pale buff appearance, but with some skins appearing to have more pink present and others more yellow. It is worth trying to produce this basic colour with your water colours and certainly a large proportion of white will be necessary in your mix.

When using ordinary cosmetics, a pink-based colour would be chosen to complement and enliven a skin which, in appearance, contains little or no warmth. Alternatively a yellow-based cream would help to tone down a skin which looks too 'ruddy'. This is not so with camouflage, where an exact colour-match should be achieved. When covering only a scarred area, the camouflage should be so perfect a match that it is indistinguishable from the surrounding skin. After camouflage has been applied it is possible to use ordinary make-up on top, when the usual 'complementary' rules of make-up can be followed. But if the patient is either a man or a child, this would be unnecessary and undesirable.

You must also consider patients who require camouflage before going on holiday. For those who tan, the original colour match could prove incorrect, so it might be sensible to suggest that they take a second colour, darker than the exact match, in the range of a cream already selected. This will enable them to cope with any darkening of the skin when this occurs. There are, however, many fair-skinned patients whose skin will not tan and who find they cannot expose themselves to direct sunlight at all for fear of burning; for such patients the colour change would only be very slight.

For those patients who already have a natural tan before going on holiday, it will be obvious in which direction their tan will further develop and a colour slightly deeper than their exact matching shade should be prescribed. White will then need to be added prior to the deeper tanning. As the tan deepens, less white will need to be added and the match can be controlled throughout. The camouflage will not only be hiding the scar but also protecting it from burning.

SKINS SCALE E–G

These will have far more pigment or melanin present in the dermis (see p. 72), which tends to obscure the network of blood capillaries. They are easier to camouflage than categories A–D (see colour chart, p. 104), being mainly one colour which varies slightly from one area of the body to another, but which is noticeably paler in areas where clothing has obscured the skin from direct sunlight. Probably the addition of pure white cover cream to the shade which matches the deeper pigmented areas will produce the paler shade where necessary. Scarring will sometimes cross from the light to the darker areas of skin; colour choice is simplified if the darker area is first matched and a little white added for the paler parts.

SKINS SCALE H–J

Here, colour matching becomes even simpler. The main colour is quite dense – revealing no blood capillaries. Invariably scarring on

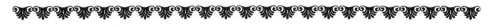

these deeper pigmented skins will have produced even darker areas. This type of skin can scar and become hyperpigmented permanently from such simple trauma as bites or stings and the scarred areas will need lightening to match the surrounding tissue.

Where skin grafting has been carried out, the same effect is produced – the graft, although taken from a matching area of the patient, will inevitably grow much darker in its new siting. Camouflage will need to be used to lighten the graft to match it to the surrounding skin.

One area where particular care must be taken when applying camouflage is on the hands. The palms are always very pale and creams applied to the back of the hands must be blended in most carefully where the colour changes so dramatically on the palm.

MATCHING COLOUR

The various manufacturers produce cover creams in a wide range of skin tones, and although some may prove to match exactly the patient's colouring, this will not always be the case. At times, when no exact match is available, you will need to mix a matching shade and there is usually a choice of ways in which you can do this.

It may be that the patient's skin colour falls midway between two shades of cream. Then if the two shades are mixed together in equal quantities, a perfect colour match will be produced and this will be a simple procedure for the patient thereafter.

However, it may be that the skin colour is slightly closer to one shade, although still lying between two available ones, and that the mix required needs to contain two parts of the closer colour to one part of the alternative. It is when no exact match is available that the knowledge of mixing colours becomes invaluable. Some specific examples may prove helpful to you.

Middle East countries tend to produce a skin colour (scale G) which can be exactly matched by using Covermark Number 1, but depending on the lifestyle of the patient, the skin may appear to have a copper tone present. Covermark Number 1 on its own, although a reasonably good match, can be adapted by one of two methods. Either a small amount of Covermark Number 8 can be added and premixed before application, or Keromask Chestnut (No. 7) can be used very sparingly as a tint over a base of Covermark Number 1 which has been applied, but not set (see Chapter 6), on the affected area. Both methods should be tried, perhaps each covering half of the scarred area, to allow comparison. Of the two creams Keromask has a slightly thinner consistency than Covermark, producing a less dense result and this could be more satisfactory to the patient. Remember that it is the patient who needs to be happy with the final result, not the cosmetician.

Another example of the choice of creams depending a great deal on the desired effect is in the case of Libyan skin (scale I), which is very dark indeed, of a rather matt or flat appearance. A mixture of Covermark Number 8 and Number 3 can be the answer here, but Keromask Chestnut (No. 7) and Umber (No. 8) should also be tried – with sometimes a small amount of white added to help simulate the matt appearance. An exact matching shade may be available without mixing, such as Dermacolor D15 or D16, or a mix of the two shades together might give the right result.

There is no doubt that the greater the variety of cover creams you use, the easier it will be to find the exact matching skin colour. Each manufacturer produces creams which react differently on different people – therefore, the more variety you have with you in your kit, the more likely you are to be able to give an excellent service.

With skin colouring in category F the Veil Number 3 might prove dark enough and is worth considering, although this sometimes appears slightly grey on the skin. Keromask Yellow (No. 5) or Veil Yellow used sparingly over the initial cover of Veil Number 3 may bring it up to an exact match.

It is essential always to look for the underlying colour of the skin when choosing the shade of cover cream. Almost always this will prove to be yellow or chestnut, even in tones A–D skin – particularly when it has been exposed to sunlight during a good summer or after a holiday abroad. Recently, with the advent of sunbeds, more and more patients whose skin tone is normally C or D are appearing with deeply tanned skins, where the basic shade of chestnut is most obvious.

People from countries situated on or near the Equator have an underlying skin colour which is difficult to detect. In almost all these patients, and particularly those who originate from the Caribbean (for example, Trinidad, Tobago and Barbados), cream that appears to be a perfect skin match will take on a grey hue when applied to the skin. This problem can easily be corrected by the addition of a very little Keromask Rose (No. 4) to the chosen shade, after application but before setting. This is a tip well worth noting, which could save you hours of frustration.

There are no generalisations that can be made about skin colour – individuals within any racial group will naturally have different skin colours. Therefore no specific formula can be given either for particular types of scarring or for particular colours of skin, and each patient must be assessed individually.

In order to mix the various colours together consistently, it will be necessary to use a constant measure for each constituent colour. For testing, only very small amounts need be used until the correct mix is found. An orange stick can be ideal as a basic measure.

If you cover exactly the flat end of the orange stick with cream and use this as one measure – or one part of the mix – tiny amounts of cream can be blended together in the palm of the hand until the correct colour is produced. Using small quantities like this will ensure less waste of cover cream.

Having mixed the small amount of cream necessary to test on the skin, place just a little *beside* the scarred area. If the match is perfect, then proceed to try a little on the scar itself. Should the scar be deeply pigmented, the matching skin colour might initially, after the application of only one thin coat, seem incorrect because the discolouration is showing through a little. In such cases if you apply a first thin coat and set it, and then a second thin coat over the first, you will usually get an exact colour match because the discolouration underneath is obliterated.

Methods of application are given in more detail in the next chapter.

6

Methods of application

The ways in which the visible effects of scarring can be improved are many and various, and you will find that there is no instant formula that can be specified for any particular condition. You will therefore have to develop your own technique so that you can achieve the best results. With each patient there will have to be careful consideration of the depth of the discolouration, together with the surrounding normal skin to be matched. There may be no exact skin colour match in the range of creams chosen as being most suitable for the skin texture, in which case you would need to blend together several colours to achieve the right shade.

After application, the cover cream should be indistinguishable from the surrounding normal skin, thus making it unnecessary for the patient to use ordinary make-up over the top of it except from personal choice. This particular consideration refers to scarring of the face, remembering that the tendency today is to wear little or no make-up, except on the eyes and lips. Therefore the final result from camouflage needs to be a natural look and certainly not one showing a thick powdered appearance which would not normally be associated with the wearer. This is particularly important when the patient is a man or a child.

Before any cover cream is applied, the area to be treated must be thoroughly cleansed to remove all the dirt or grease which could cause the cover to 'slide' on application.

You will find that the different methods you use to apply creams can affect the end result, simply because of the differences you will come across in basic skin types and textures. Details of the methods available are given later in this chapter. However, no matter which method of application proves most suitable for the type of skin you are treating, all cover creams must be applied very sparingly for two reasons: firstly a more natural look can be expected and this is less likely to be noticeable; secondly the cream will be less likely to rub off on to clothes. Although one very thin coat of cream may not be dense enough to obliterate a scar, rather than

applying a thick coat initially, a better end result will be obtained if a second or even a third thin application is added over the original, should this prove necessary. As a general rule, each thin application or coat should be set by means of talcum powder, a colourless translucent powder or the setting powder produced especially for the purpose by some manufacturers of cover cream.

So, without exception, cover creams must be applied sparingly. One thin coat may prove sufficient but if necessary, subsequent thin coats – each being set after application – can be added possibly just on small parts of the original area where the scarring is still visible.

The exception to the rule of setting each separate coat of cover cream, as it is applied, will be where an additional cream is added to the basic shade after it has been applied to the skin, in order to change this shade slightly to tone in with the surrounding tissue. This would be the case, for instance, when adding a toner to a cheek to simulate the flushed appearance of the opposite side of the face. So that the toner will blend easily with the cover cream, it should be added before the cream has been set.

For a while after application, cover creams tend to 'sit on top' of the skin but within an hour they will be absorbed slightly into the skin and become almost impossible to detect. From this time onwards the creams will be stable. Although more difficult to remove than ordinary cosmetics, cover cream can be rubbed off immediately after application – especially before setting has been completed and sometimes 'impatient' patients will need to be restrained from doing this!

The thin coating of cover cream having been applied, the next step is to proceed with a liberal application of setting powder using a dry piece of cotton wool as an applicator, and making sure not to miss any area where cream has been placed. The excess powder should then be lightly and gently brushed off in a downward direc- tion, either with a soft brush or dry cotton wool. Finally blot the area with damp cotton wool. This will have the effect of removing any obvious traces of powder and also help to set the camouflage more efficiently. This entire procedure should be followed for each coat of cover cream that is applied, but it can be followed in three different ways.

Each of these three different methods of setting can be recom- mended but the third method is the one most likely to be adopted by busy patients. The methods are:

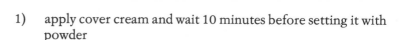

1) apply cover cream and wait 10 minutes before setting it with powder

2) apply cover cream and set immediately but wait 10 minutes before brushing off excess powder and blotting

3) apply cover cream, then powder; brush off excess and blot immediately with a damp cotton wool swab.

Each of these methods is worth trying to see which gives the best result, for what proves right in one case may not necessarily be so in another.

When the camouflage needs to be removed it can be rubbed with any kind of cream such as a cleanser, a cold cream or one of the removal creams supplied by the manufacturers for the purpose. The thicker the original cover, the more difficult it will be to dislodge, but the cleanser will gradually soften the camouflage, which can then be wiped away completely with a piece of dampened cotton wool. It is the oil present in the removal cream which dislodges the camouflage.

A point worth noting is that water-dampened cotton wool is the most absorbent material for removing anything greasy from the skin. Soft paper tissues are not so efficient and, because they contain resin, can cause allergic reactions in some patients.

METHODS OF APPLICATION

Having discussed the amount of cream for each application, we can now look at the equally important question of how it is applied, because different methods produce different results.

There are three ways in which the creams can be applied:

1) with a brush
2) with a dampened natural cosmetic sponge
3) with the finger.

With a brush

Where the scar is of the thin hairline type (a), a finger would be too wide for applying cream and could spread it over too large an area. Remember that the camouflage should only cover the actual scar, and therefore in this instance should be applied thinly by brush, up to the inside edges of the scar (b). Then tap lightly with the middle finger (c) where the cream has been applied, to blur the hard edge of the cream and blend it into the surrounding skin. The middle finger is the best one to use in this instance, as one tends to press too hard with the index finger and not only might this hurt the patient but it could also remove some of the cream. An alternative to tapping with the finger, particularly where the scar is tender, is to press gently and slightly turn the finger on contact, which will have the same effect – spreading the edges of the camouflage to blend it in. When the cream is blended in, powder (d) and blot with damp cotton wool (e).

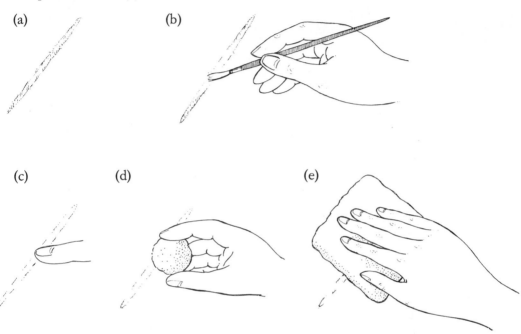

(a)

(b)

(c)

(d)

(e)

With a dampened natural cosmetic sponge

Natural cosmetic sponges are available from many chemists and stores. They are very small, being only about half the size of a thumb, and have tiny perforations all over them. Pieces cut from larger natural sponges are less manageable and unsuitable for this work because their perforations are too large.

First immerse the sponge in water to soften it, then squeeze it gently to remove excess water and leave it just damp. Now take some of the required cover cream in the palm of your hand and press the damp sponge into it. The sponge is now loaded and ready for use on the patient.

The cosmetician loads the sponge in this way for reasons of cleanliness so that she will not re-load the sponge from the pot, running the risk of cross-infection between patients, whereas the patient can load his or her own sponge from the pot without first taking some cream into the palm of his or her hand. In either case it is wise to test the amount on the sponge by first pressing the sponge on to the back of your hand before applying it to the scarred area.

Cover cream applied by this method will be found to give only a very light covering, which is excellent for toning down conditions such as rosacea, or a very red nose. By only lightly covering these conditions, allowing some of the skin colour to show through, a natural effect is obtained, whereas a dense cover would look completely unnatural. Sponge application can in some cases be the best method for covering bruising, although when deep hyperpigmentation is present, the cover obtained by sponge application can be insufficient.

After sponge application, use of the finger should not be necessary. Should a little too much cream have been applied, simply reverse the sponge to its clean side and press gently over the creamed area to remove a little of the excess cream. When the result is satisfactory, powdering and blotting can be done in the usual way. If a second coating of cream is necessary, this can be applied successfully in the same way.

With the finger

This can be done in one of three ways. Firstly by a simple rubbing action; secondly by pressing gently and turning the finger on the spot (using the middle finger); or thirdly, if no soreness or bruising is present, by a gentle tapping movement, again with the middle finger. All three ways can be equally successful and give good coverage. Each should be tried to see which produces the best result.

Where a large area of scarring is involved, a rubbing movement will be quickest and when this produces good results, it would be the method to choose. Whichever method is chosen, however, the cover cream should be applied to the scarred area only, and extended to the edges by finger pressure before being powdered and blotted in the usual way. Camouflage can be spoiled if you extend with the cover cream the area of apparent scarring by even a small amount because unless the normal surrounding skin is of a uniform colour, this could mean much more correcting work for the patient to match the camouflage to the normal skin. However, skin rarely is one colour; colour differences are almost always present in the normal skin, caused for example by broken veins, dark shadows or freckles. These imperfections will need to be

matched on the camouflage area in order to obtain a natural finish and this is particularly important, of course, on the face.

MATCHING IMPERFECTIONS (FAKING FAULTS)

Hiding broken veins

Most female patients will prefer that obvious broken veins be obliterated by camouflage, on the unscarred as well as the scarred areas. This should be done in the following way:

1) match the cover cream to the basic skin colour
2) apply to the scarred area by the chosen method of application until the scar is obliterated
3) set the camouflage and blot
4) place a small amount of the matching camouflage cream in the palm of your hand, spreading it to cover an area of about 3 square centimetres
5) press a dampened cosmetic sponge into the cream on your palm loading it thinly on one side only
6) test it on the back of your hand
7) roll the creamed side of the sponge gently over the non-camouflaged veined area until the discolouration is hidden
8) turn the sponge to its clean side and blot the area until an absolutely natural finish has been achieved
9) set with finishing powder
10) blot with damp cotton wool.

Matching broken veins

Method for patients with natural high facial colouring which needs to be matched after camouflage (used particularly for men and children):

1) match the cover cream to the basic skin colour
2) apply to scarred area until the scar is obliterated
3) do not set with powder yet
4) press a dampened cosmetic sponge once into one of the pink toning creams
5) now press the same sponge once on to any cream-based navy blue coloured eyeshadow
6) press once more on to the pink toning cream (thus making a kind of sandwich of the two colours)
7) test the depth of colour on the back of your hand
8) press gently – by a rolling action – on top of the cover cream already applied to the area of scarring; two or three rolling

movements may be needed to cover all the area being treated, to match the corresponding normal area

9)   set with finishing powder
10) blot with dampened cotton wool

Matching dark areas of shadow around the eyes

Method to be used when camouflage has hidden the natural colouring particularly for men:

1)   match the cream to the basic skin colour
2)   apply to scarred area until the scar is obliterated
3)   set the camouflage and blot
4)   choose a cream to match the darkened areas around the eyes
5)   load a dampened sponge with the darker cream chosen
6)   ask the patient to keep his eyes open but to look up at the ceiling
7)   gently roll the sponge right up to the lashes of the lower eyelid, matching the depth of colour on the opposite side

If the darkened colouring also stretches up into the eye socket:

8)   ask the patient to close his eyes
9)   exert finger control on eyelid – one finger lifting the brow, another pulling the eyelid outwards to remove skin creases
10) apply loaded sponge to the upper eyelid until the depth of the colour is correctly matching the opposite eye
11) apply finishing powder over the whole area
12) blot with damp cotton wool

Matching 5 o'clock shadow on partial missing beard area

1)   match cream to the basic skin colour
2)   apply cover cream to scarred area
3)   set and blot
4)   match the colour of existing beard or stubble (Covermark provide a grey toner for this purpose; alternatively black and white can be mixed together and a coloured toner added to the mix if necessary)
5)   load a damp sponge with a *little* of the matched stubble colour
6)   gently roll this across the chin until the camouflage resembles the rest of the natural stubble
7)   apply finishing powder and dust off
8)   blot with damp cotton wool

Note if faults need to be simulated on any areas of the body after camouflage, you should always use a damp sponge as an applicator except in the case of freckles.

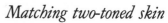

Matching two-toned skin

Sponge application can also be used when the skin tone appears to have two basic shades, possibly caused by the partial tanning of a fair skin. The following procedure should then be used for successful camouflage:

1)   match the cream to the basic skin tone
2)   cover the scarred area completely with this shade
3)   match the darker skin tone
4)   load a damp sponge with the darker shade
5)   apply sparingly over the original pale camouflage, leaving the first colour to show through partially
6)   apply finishing powder and brush off
7)   blot with dampened cotton wool

Matching freckles

1)   match the cream to the basic skin tone
2)   cover scarred area completely
3)   apply setting powder and dust off
4)   blot with dampened cotton wool
5)   match freckle colour
6)   with a fine brush, simulate freckles with small spots of freckle colour over the whole area
7)   apply finishing powder and dust off
8)   blot with damp cotton wool.

Note that in some cases a better result is obtained by applying basic skin colour and simulating freckles prior to using setting powder.

EYEBROWS

In some cases a whole eyebrow or part of an eyebrow may be missing and this may be only a temporary defect, before a hair bearing graft is given. It may be possible for a false matching eyebrow to be made (see Chapter 10, *Prosthetics*). However, it is sometimes possible, particularly with women and children, to use an eyebrow pencil to simulate the existing eyebrow. Take care when choosing the colour of the pencil, because brown pencil tends to look a rather ginger shade when applied to the skin and black can appear harsh. You will find that a grey pencil will give a remarkably natural appearance for any fair-haired patient, including those with auburn tints, as well as being the obvious choice for patients with grey or white hair.

Grey pencil can also be used in conjunction with either brown or black because the combination of two colours will give a good natural appearance. Remember never to draw a single line to simulate an eyebrow, or use strokes all in one direction. If you use a combination of grey and one other colour you should start with the grey pencil, drawing in tiny hairs at right-angles to the direction of natural growth (a). Follow this with the main colour drawn with tiny strokes in the correct line of growth (b).

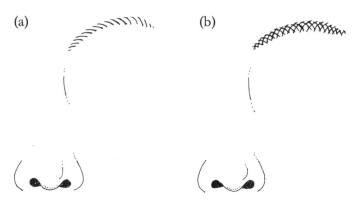

In this way you will get a good balance. A useful maxim when using eyebrow pencil is 'if in doubt, use grey'.

COVERING BRUISING, TATTOOS OR DEEPLY PIGMENTED SCARS

These types of scarring can be difficult to camouflage well but recent additions to the range of cover creams have helped to solve the problem.

Tattoos

Before using the skin matching shade, try a first coat as follows, setting it firmly with powder. Use a brush as applicator and carefully colour out the dyes which might otherwise show through the finished camouflage. Over blue tattoos use Dermacolor D32 or Veil Rose. Over red tattoos use Dermacolor 1742 or Veil Olive.

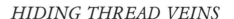
These occur particularly on the thighs and lower areas of the legs. The best disguise comes from applying a first coat of either pure white, Veil Olive, or Dermacolor D0 or 1742, using a small brush to trace the outline of each vein. This can be a tedious task but, remembering that cover creams can be expected to last at least several days on the body, it is not one which needs to be carried out daily. The tracing should be set with powder and blotted before you apply the main skin-matching shade, again tracing with a brush. Finally tap in with the middle finger before setting with powder and blotting. If any parts of the vein still show through, you may need to touch out these small areas again with the brush containing the skin-matching shade, and then set and blot them. Excellent results can be obtained this way.

CAMOUFLAGE ON THE LOWER LEG, FROM KNEE TO ANKLE

For some reason, camouflage on the lower leg can look perfect to anyone seeing it from the front, but to the patient seeing it from above, it can appear as a bad skin match with powder over it.

However, you can overcome this problem, after you have camouflaged the actual scar, by adding a very thin patchy coat of the skin shade all over the leg from the foot to the knee. This is best done by pressing small patches of matching cream at say 2 or 3 cm intervals, using very little cream and then spreading this over the whole area by rubbing. In this way the natural skin colour will not be obscured and a perfectly natural finish will be seen not only from the front but also from the patient's-eye view. Naturally you will have to treat the other leg in the same way, to give both legs the same appearance.

INDENTED (ATROPHIC), PROTRUDING (HYPERTROPHIC) AND KELOID SCARS

These are probably the most difficult types of scarring to camouflage successfully, the scars not being level with the surrounding skin. Flaps and grafts are particularly difficult. Where these scars are either hypopigmented or hyperpigmented (see p. 96), camouflage will make a definite improvement, as it will disguise

the discolouration, but the appearance can sometimes be further improved by subtle use of colour round the edge of the scar using a highlighting and/or shading process.

Pale shades are known as highlighters, and dark ones are shaders. When a highlighter is applied to any area it will give the effect of bringing it forward, making it appear to protrude and look larger. The opposite happens when shaders are applied, giving a sunken or smaller appearance. From this you might think that applying a shade slightly paler than the perfect skin match, all over a sunken scar, would make it appear level but this rarely happens, and nor does a darker shade make a raised scar look flatter, although it is worth trying highlighting or shading in the first instance. However, if you cover the scar with the exact skin-matching shade, you can then try to improve the finish in the following ways.

Indented (atrophic) scars

1) Take a shade of cream slightly paler than the matching skin shade and use a small brush to apply a thin band – about 3 mm wide – around the *inside* edge of the scar. Tap it in with the finger tip and set in the usual way (a).
2) Alternatively, using a slightly darker cream than the matching skin shade and with a small brush, apply a thin band – about 3 mm wide – immediately *outside* the actual scar. Blend it in by lightly tapping with the finger and set in the usual way (b).
3) Try 1 and 2 together (c).

(a)

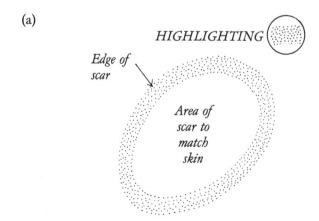

HIGHLIGHTING

Edge of scar

Area of scar to match skin

(b)

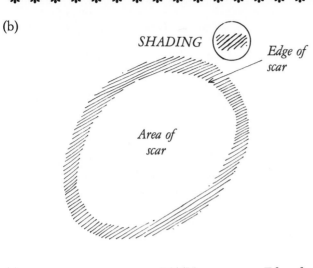

SHADING

Edge of
scar

Area of
scar

(c)

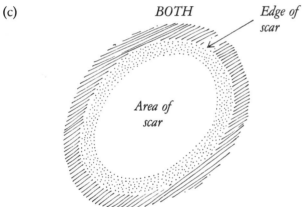

BOTH

Edge of
scar

Area of
scar

By highlighting and shading processes you are attempting to make
the scarred area appear less indented and the surrounding area
less protruding.

Protruding (hypertrophic) scars

The procedure for these types of scar needs to be the exact
opposite of that for atrophic scars:

1)   With a shade of cream slightly darker than the matching skin
     shade, use a small brush to draw a band – about 3 mm wide
     – on the *inside* edge of the scar. Tap it with a finger to blend
     and set in the usual way (a).
2)   With a lighter shade of cream, use a brush to apply a 3 mm

band immediately *outside* the edge of the scar, on the normal flat skin. Tap in with a finger and set as usual (b).

3) Try 1 and 2 together (c).

(a)

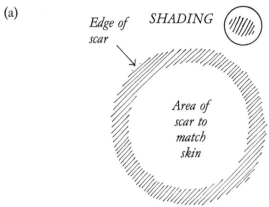

Edge of scar

SHADING

Area of scar to match skin

(b)

HIGHLIGHTING

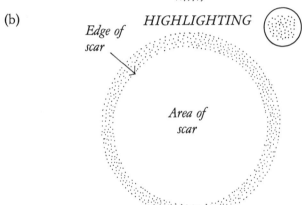

Edge of scar

Area of scar

(c)

BOTH

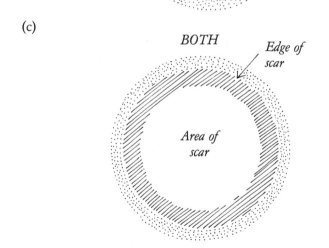

Edge of scar

Area of scar

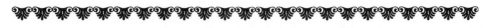

Scars will react differently to this treatment; sometimes there will be no appreciable difference, making it a pointless operation for the patient, but at other times results can be superb.

Keloid scars (See Chapter 11, *Medical Terminology,* for explanation)

It is unlikely that highlighting and shading can improve a simple camouflage on this type of scarring. Usually the best you can do is to hide the discolouration, using a small brush to spread the cover cream on the puckered areas not reached by finger application. Aim at an improvement, but you cannot expect obliteration. Keloid scars can successfully be given medical treatment and will then be much easier to conceal with camouflage. Dermacolor 406 used as a first coat before camouflage will improve the end result.

DROPPED OUTLINE OF MOUTH

A noticeable dropping and loss of contour around the mouth, sometimes producing the appearance of a sneer, can be caused by various conditions such as grafting or can follow a stroke. It may be possible to improve the appearance with surgery, for example a 'muscle sling', but even patients who can be helped in this way, may have an interim period of some months when help through camouflage will be appreciated. Although cosmetic camouflage cannot physically change this condition, it can improve the appearance considerably. The following method is suggested:

1) match cream to the basic skin colouring around the mouth (a)
2) apply a little of the cover cream over the drooping area (b)
3) set the cover cream and blot it
4) take a lip pencil and draw a line of contour exactly matching the unaffected side (c)
5) using a pale and preferably pearlised lipstick, apply with a brush within the line drawn, filling in the whole lip area (d)
6) get the patient to 'blot' her lips on a paper tissue.

Note A pearlised lipstick is suggested because, as this can be termed a highlighter, it will draw people's eyes to the colour rather than to the shape of the mouth.

These suggestions for dealing with specific problems should provide a basis for treatment of any kind of scarring. It is impossible to describe every type which may need to be camouflaged, because all scars are different. However, armed with a knowledge of highlighting and shading and what is possible, you should be able to improve any scar, no matter how distorted it may have made the skin.

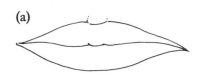

(a)

(b)

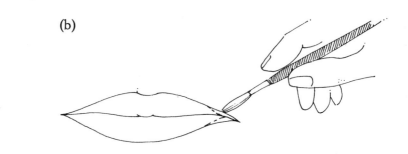

(c)

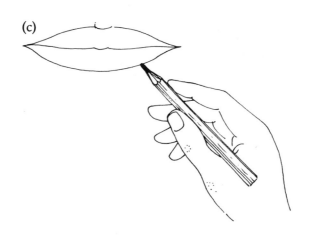

(d)

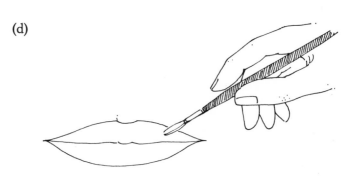

7

Finger massage for scars

The clinical cosmetician can play an important part in the improvement of scarring by advising her patients on the importance of finger massage.

Scars are produced as a result of the body's normal healing mechanism. They are a mixture of blood vessels and fibrous tissue in amounts which vary according to the age of the scar. It is perfectly normal for scars to appear extremely good at first but then to go through a period when they appear worse, becoming redder and more raised. In time they will become pale again and more flattened. This whole process may take more than twelve to eighteen months.

Scars can be greatly helped by being vigorously massaged. This reduces any tendency for the skin to become stuck to underlying structures and by encouraging the resolution of the redness and swelling it speeds the achievement of a flatter and paler scar. Application of some bland cream, which reduces the friction between the finger and the scar, is a help during vigorous massage.

In massaging the scar, it is important to use enough force to move the skin over the underlying structures. Massage should be done with the finger tips in a tight circular motion (a) working all over the scar, and giving special attention to raised edges and places where hardness can be felt. Ideally this exercise should be carried out for ten minutes, six times each day but, as this might be difficult for busy patients, you can suggest that they do the massaging while relaxing – watching TV, reading or using the telephone – but if possible one hour's massage each day should be aimed at.

Massage should begin as soon as possible after the scar has been sustained; after surgery, this means within days of the sutures being removed, and with other scars as soon as any accompanying bruising has gone. Remember, a scar which is massaged will certainly improve and may go completely but a scar left alone will almost certainly be a scar for life. Massage should be continued

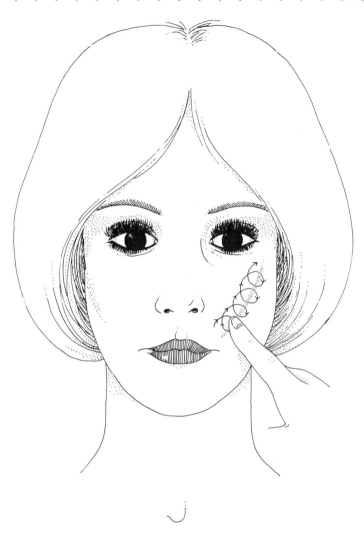

over a long period – even for months – until it is obviously no longer necessary.

Many surgeons state that no improvement can be expected from massaging a scar which is more than five years old, but massage has been tried on scars sustained many years previously and has made a noticeable improvement. Massage will certainly do no harm and is always worth trying. However, the older the scar, the longer it will take to show any improvement.

Whenever a patient arrives for treatment with scarring sustained from the skin having been cut, whether by surgery or some other trauma, one of your first tasks should be to ask whether advice has

already been given on finger massage. In some cases the patient may already have been made aware of its importance, but you will do no harm in stressing the point.

It is possible that the patient has not understood that the cream to be applied before massage is only a lubricant. In clearing up such a misunderstanding you should take the chance to give a full explanation of the improvement that regular massage can achieve, and to demonstrate the correct way to do it.

You should also make the point that any camouflage present on the scar is bound to be removed by using cream for massage. However this is a small price to pay if the scar improves and eventually disappears.

The short time taken at a consultation to explain the massage is amply repaid by the results that can be expected if the patient acts on your advice. It is better that your patients cure their scars, rather than have to use camouflage indefinitely.

8

Face shapes

Although no two faces are identical, it will be helpful if you can easily recognise the shape that most nearly matches your patient's face. If you are to correct any faults you must first assess them correctly.

An oval-shaped face is believed to be ideal, with perfect symmetry and no obvious irregularities. This is rarely found in adults, however, because even in the late teens, muscles begin to slacken, the sides of the face start to drop and the face changes shape. This process continues throughout life and will probably cause each face-shape to alter, in its individual way, several times during a lifetime.

An understanding of these basic shapes will help you assess a face, and indicate particular areas where highlighting or shading may be added to improve the appearance. Without using a ruler you must learn to estimate the balance between width and length and first you must see the basic shape clearly by moving the hair from the face.

THE SEVEN VARIATIONS OF BASIC FACE-SHAPES

| SQUARE | ROUND | RECTANGLE |

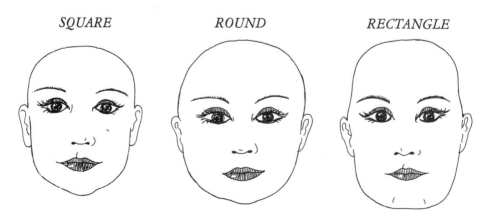

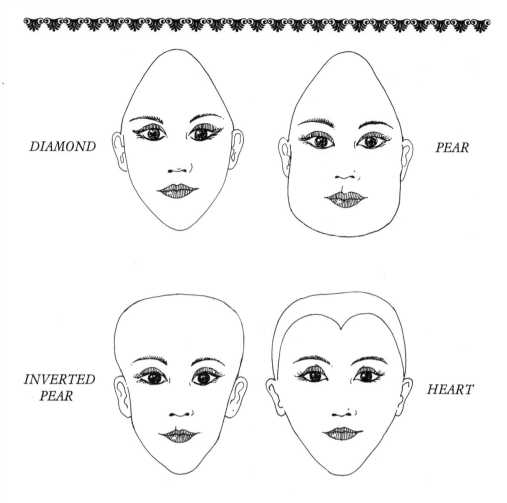

DIAMOND

PEAR

INVERTED
PEAR

HEART

ESTIMATING THE BALANCE OF A FACE

Look at the width across the wide
part of the forehead A.

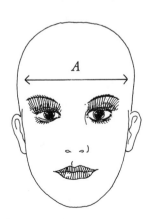

How does the width A relate to an imaginary line from the temple to the wide part of the jaw B?
Is the vertical length B greater or less than the width A, or is it the same?

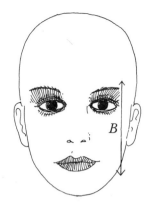

Now consider the width of the jaw at the widest part C:
Is this greater or less than the forehead width A?
Is the width C greater or less than the length B?
If these three measurements A, B and C are about the same, the face could be termed 'square' – but before deciding, consider the width across the eyes D.

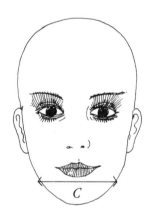

Is the face wider at the eyes D than it is across the forehead A or jaw C?
If so it can be termed 'round', as long as A, B and C are approximately equal.

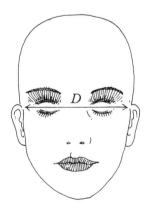

Relationship of the dimensions in the seven face-shapes

SQUARE FACE

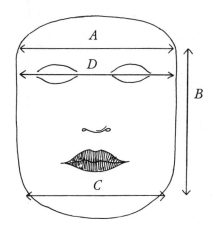

A, B, C and D are equal.

ROUND FACE

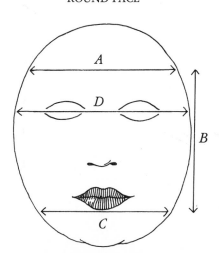

A, B and C are equal and less than D.

RECTANGULAR FACE

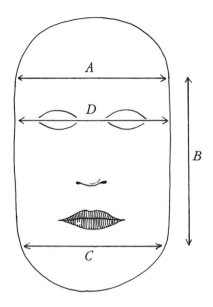

A, C and D are equal and less than B.

DIAMOND FACE

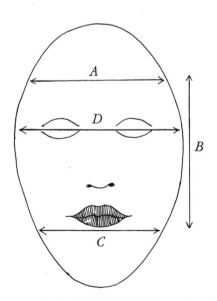

A and C are equal and less than B and D. The chin will be long and the centre hairline high.

PEAR-SHAPED FACE

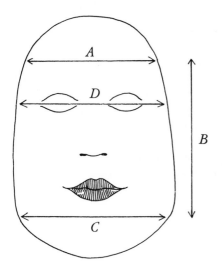

The narrowest part is across the fore-head line A with increasing width at D and C (eyes and jaw); B can vary but will usually be about the same as the jaw width C.

INVERTED PEAR-SHAPED FACE

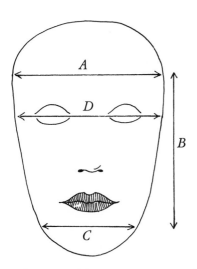

The widest part is the forehead line A with decreasing width at D and C (eyes and jaw). B is approximately the same as the forehead width A.

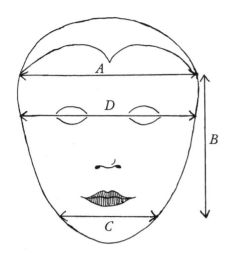

The widest part is the forehead A with the eye line D only slightly narrower. The narrowest part is the jawline C with B approximately the same as the eye line D. The central hairline is dipped on to the forehead, with what is often called a widow's peak.

With practice you will soon recognise these seven face-shapes easily, and will probably find the rectangular shape is the most common, for a simple reason. The skin from the temples and sides of the cheeks is the first to show signs of ageing and sagging, so that the skin around the jawline becomes heavier. This undoubtedly causes an oval face to become more rectangular, and the same applies to some extent in the case of the diamond, the square and the heart-shaped faces.

The ability to recognise face shapes is important if you are working as a clinical cosmetician, because you will be concerned with the correction of 'faults' which may have occurred in such cases as strokes, road traffic accidents, facial grafts and so on. A knowledge of highlighting and shading will be essential – highlighting to emphasise good points and shading to help to conceal the bad ones. (See also Chapter 6, *Methods of Application.*)

To highlight an area you need to use only white or light colours, – such as 'pearlised' products – which reflect light easily. The reflective quality of all pale shades makes things appear larger, rounder and more prominent. For instance, a highlighter applied to the areas under the eyes, where deep shadows are apparent, makes the eyes appear less sunken and therefore younger, larger and brighter. This, in turn, draws attention to the colour of the eyes, and you can emphasise this good point by blending a little matching eyeshadow on to the lids.

Colours which do not reflect light are used for shaders and will give an illusion of hollowness and depth when applied to the skin. Shaders can be brown, deep blue or the darker greys, and can for instance be used to create shadow on an over-prominent area above an eye – on the part which tends to 'droop' and overhang the eye. Shading, used sparingly over this prominent area, reduces the prominence considerably. In the same way heavy or enlarged lids can look more delicate with shading. Surprisingly, many people make the mistake of using light colours such as pink or lilac on heavy lids, which only enlarges them and presents an unbalanced appearance.

As a clinical cosmetician you should never encourage patients to use certain colours simply because they are in fashion, unless that particular fashion provides the improvement the patient needs. Although camouflage does not normally include ordinary make-up, you will have some conditions to treat where the application of highlighting and/or shading, with perhaps the introduction of eyeshadow or lipstick, will be just what is needed to complete the camouflage you have applied.

A patient may be suffering from more than one problem as the result of an accident. There may be a scar crossing the cheek and eyelid which has healed unevenly, so that one side of the scar appears fatter or more prominent than the other, on both cheek and eyelid. In this case the first priority is to match the skin tone and apply camouflage to the actual scar. After this, the principles of highlighting and shading can be applied by using a slightly deeper shade of cover cream to the bloated or enlarged area and making the sunken side a little paler, thus achieving a balanced finish. If only one side of the scar is irregular, say by being enlarged, then you will only need to shade that part, and can leave the normal side untouched.

Female patients, particularly, will be grateful for advice on complementary make-up after camouflage. For that reason and because it can be of benefit to the patient, the next section discusses various corrective measures which can be used with make-up, and the principles behind them which can be useful when you deal with areas of scarring.

REMEDIAL TREATMENT: MAKE-UP

Whenever you are applying make-up, you should consider it carefully in the context of the shape of the face and the prominent features such as the eyes and nose. Merely to follow current fashion for every face regardless of its good or bad features will give you bad results in ninety-nine cases out of every hundred. Make-up should complement the face and not change it out of all recognition.

In this section for the shaders and highlighters mentioned, you should use dark or light shades of camouflage creams. Ordinary make-up bases or sticks of highlighters and shaders can however be substituted when your only concern is the application of make-up to complement facial features and achieve a natural, balanced appearance.

Forehead

Make-up bases should never be applied right up to the hairline; instead spread the cream to about 15 mm from it and then use the sides of your hands, to 'stretch' the base to the hairline. This prevents the creams from marking the hair.

Feature to be corrected	*Application*
(a) Forehead overlarge compared with the rest of the face (inverted-pear type) 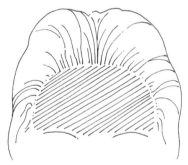	(a) On the forehead use a shade of foundation darker than the one on the rest of the face.
(b) Hairline low, forehead small 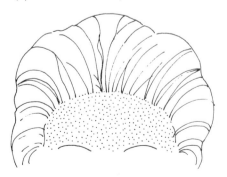	(b) On the forehead use a shade of foundation lighter than the one for the rest of the face.

Feature to be corrected	Application
(c) Centre of forehead prominent with sides receding	(c) Using shades of foundation darker and lighter than the main shade for the face, apply the darker shade in the centre of the forehead and blend it with the lighter one at the sides.

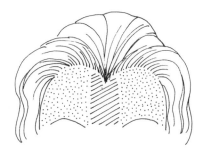

KEY

 Dark Foundation

 Light Foundation

Eyes

First you must consider the set of the eyes. Ideally the space between the eyes should be at least as wide as one eye. The perfectly proportioned eye line contains the width of five eyes, with one eye width outside each eye and one between them. If there is less than one eye width between the eyes they are said to be too close-set and you can use make-up to correct this appearance. On the other hand, having the width between the eyes slightly larger than the width of one eye is often attractive and there is no need for correction.

Having determined the set of the eyes, your next step is to explore the use of highlighters and shaders.

Feature to be corrected	Application
(a) Close-set eyes	(a) Highlight inside inner corners, to give impression of eyes being further apart.

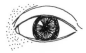

Feature to be corrected	Application
(b) Small eyes	(b) Highlight around the outer corners to give an impression of width.
(c) Bulbous eyes with overhanging brows 	(c) Use dark shader (or eyeshadow) on lids; use dark shader (or eyeshadow) immediately above; use highlighter above to 'lift', blending all these together where they meet.
(d) droopy eyes 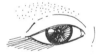	(d) Highlight area above eyes as illustrated, but use shader on outside corners. The highlight will draw attention to the area above the eyes and the shader will take attention away from the droop.

KEY

 Highlighter

 Shader

Shaders and highlighters in the brown, beige and cream coloured ranges used as described give good natural results on younger faces.

The same principles can be applied to improving older faces, but you should use highlighters and shaders which also add a little colour, such as light and dark blues or grey/greens.

Many eyeshadows are available in sets of various shades of one basic colour. When choosing the most suitable colour for a patient you should take into account the clothes being worn and the colour of the eyes.

Eyeliners are a type of shader and can greatly enhance the appearance of the eyes. You should never encircle an eye with eyeliner because this gives a 'piggy-eyed' look, making the eyes appear much smaller than they really are (d). If you apply eyeliner to both top and bottom lids, the lines should not be allowed to meet at the corners (a). It is preferable however to apply liners only to the upper lids (c), or to the upper lids together with only the *outer half* of the lower lids (b).

I recommend that you never use a black eyeliner as the colour is too harsh. Apply liners with a very thin brush, resting it half on the lid and half on the lashes, so that no skin is left bare between them, and fading the line away on the outer edges so that there is no abrupt end.

Correct eyeliner application   *Incorrect eyeliner application*

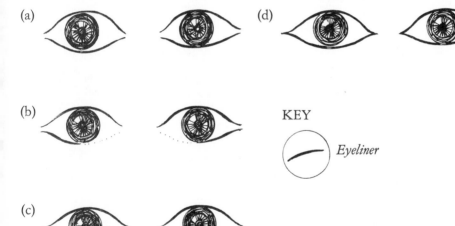

(a)

(d)

(b)

KEY

Eyeliner

(c)

If a patient has been burned, the eyelashes may have been destroyed permanently. While, with practice, some people attach false lashes to the eyelid (see Chapter 10, *Prosthetics*), it is a difficult task for a patient to tackle each day. With no existing lashes as support, the false ones can slip and cause the wearer embarrassment. As an alternative you can apply eyeliner discreetly along the edge of the lid, giving it definition in the same way that lashes do, and adding expression to the eyes to subdue the otherwise blank look. The result is usually best if you treat the top lid only. (See Chapter 10, *Prosthetics* for more information on the grafting of eyelashes.)

Feature to be corrected	*Application*
(a) Thick-edged lids	(a) Use shader along the edge of the upper lid and highlighter on the rest of the lid – blending them together where they meet.

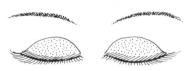

(b(i)) Lids which do not show when the eyes are open	(b(i)) Use highlighter or pearlised eyeshadow on whole of the upper lid with eyeliner along the top lid only.

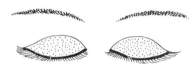

(b(ii))	(b(ii)) In addition to b(i), highlighter can be used to enlarge the eyes. Apply round the outside edge, and under the eye up to half the eye width in. *Note* This is not recommended when the upper eyelid has a downward droop on the outer corner, when it would only highlight the droop.

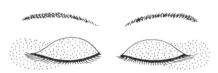

KEY

 Highlighter

 Shader

 Eyeliner

Correction may be necessary to the shape of the nose, for although the profile cannot be changed with camouflage, the frontal appearance can be improved by skilful application of shaders and highlighters.

COMPARING THE LENGTH OF THE NOSE WITH THE PROPORTIONS
OF THE REST OF THE FACE.

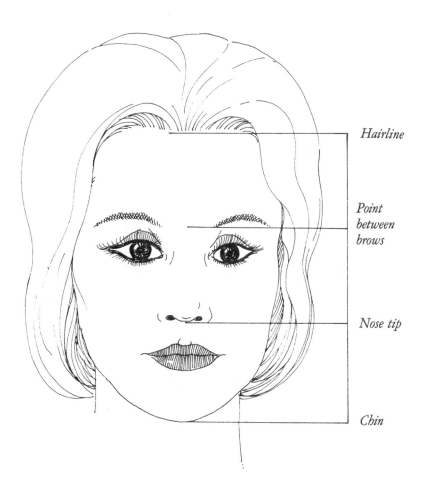

Hairline

Point
between
brows

Nose tip

Chin

For the ideal face the three sections as shown should be approximately equal.

Feature to be corrected	*Application*
(a) Fat or wide nose 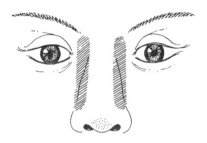	(a) Apply shader in parallel lines on each side up to eyebrows. Apply a highlight to tip if the nose needs lengthening (only place the shader up to the eyebrows if the length is right, if too long refer to diagram (b).
(b) Long nose 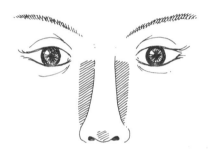	(b) Apply shader to tip of nose and add parallel lines of shader on each side, close to – but not on – the nose, up to the corners of the eyes.
(c) Thin nose 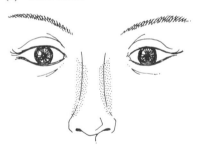	(c) Use highlighter on both sides of the nose up to the eye level.
(d) Bulbous-ended nose 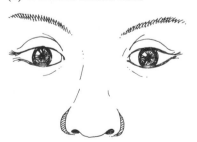	(d) Use shader on both sides at base.

KEY

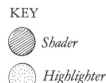

Shader

Highlighter

It is unwise to highlight the bridge of the nose, because under lights or in sunlight the make-up will reflect and the nose will become too apparent.

Cheeks

Rouge or blusher can be applied to improve the contours and to draw the viewer's eyes to colour rather than shape. Heavy areas can be broken up with a little carefully placed colour used as a highlighter.

Correct positioning is shown below on the basis of face shapes, but note that you should never apply rouge or blusher right up to the nose.

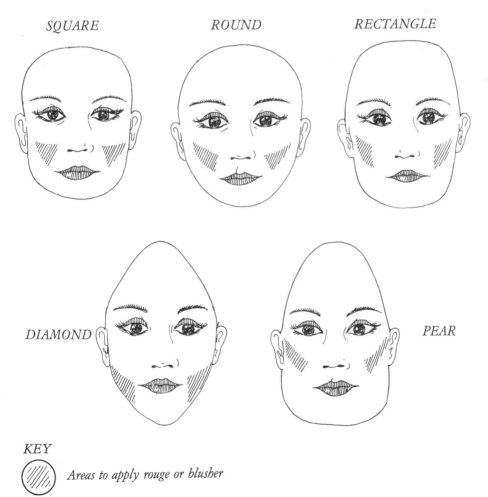

SQUARE   *ROUND*   *RECTANGLE*

DIAMOND   *PEAR*

KEY

Areas to apply rouge or blusher

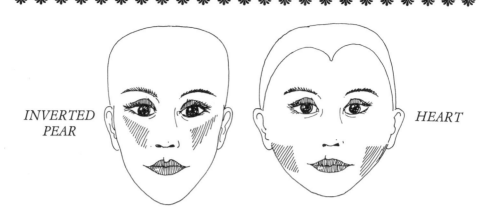

INVERTED
PEAR

HEART

Lips

Feature to be corrected

(a) Small upper lip

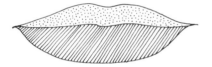

(b) Large upper lip

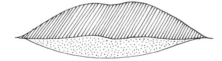

Application

(a) Apply light shade of lipstick to upper lip.
Add darker shade to lower lip.

(b) Apply dark shade of lipstick on top lip. Apply paler shade of lipstick on lower lip.

(See also Chapter 6, *Methods of Application,* for information on lips affected by scarring due to trauma.)

Chins

Feature to be corrected

(a) Heavy jawline

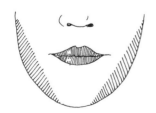

Application

(a) Apply a dark shade of foundation or a shader to this area to reduce heaviness.

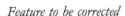

Feature to be corrected	Application
(b) Protruding chin	(b) Add shader across the area indicated.

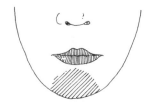

(c) Small chin	(c) Enlarge the appearance with a highlighter or pale shade of foundation.

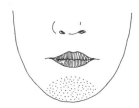

REMEDIAL TREATMENT: GROOMING

Eyebrows

If you need to tidy up the eyebrows, always pluck the hairs in the direction of the growth, and mainly from under the brow line. Occasionally a few stray hairs need to be removed from the centre between the brows. A touch of cold cream or cleansing cream on the brows before starting makes the plucking much easier and you can take away any stinging by applying a cold damp pad afterwards.

A variety of eyebrow-plucking instruments is available, ranging from long thin pointed ones (a) to some which have a spring attached and are referred to as automatic. However, the easiest sort to manipulate – without causing pain – are those shaped like bent scissors (b).

(a)

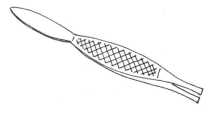

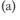

(b)

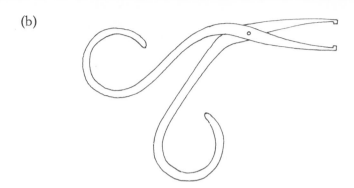

These (b) can be laid flat on to the skin and do not obscure your line of vision while you are working. Lift one hair at a time into the gripper, then lift the brow and press gently on to the brow bone; extract the hair by pulling gently sideways. The pressure on the brow deadens the nerve momentarily so the extraction can be painless.

Eyebrows may need shaping where they have been formed by a hair-bearing graft.

To find the correct width for an eyebrow, place a pencil to touch the side of the base of the nose and the outside corner of the eye; the eyebrow should terminate where it touches the pencil.

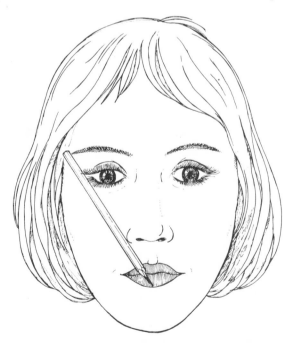

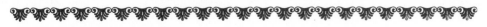

Stray hairs beyond this ideal point of termination will need to be removed. In older women you will find that the outside edges of the brows drop considerably as the face muscles slacken. If the brows are left unplucked the expression appears downcast or depressed, and the appearance is spoiled.

If you wear spectacles for close work you may have difficulty plucking your own eyebrows. This can be overcome by wearing your spectacles upsidedown temporarily. Alternatively, you can get a special type of spectacles which have been designed to overcome this problem by having hinged lenses that can be moved up and down. Otherwise you can use a magnifying mirror or a magnifying glass.

Eyebrow plucking can make an enormous improvement to the appearance and give your patients a younger look. Carried out correctly, it need not be the painful process that is often expected. (See also Chapter 10, *Prosthetics*.)

Eyebrows and eyelashes: loss of colour

There can be a total loss or partial loss of colour to the lashes and brows, particularly in the condition called vitiligo, which is, unfortunately, permanent: individual hairs can lose all colour and look pure white. While mascara can be applied to either lashes or brows to improve the appearance, it cannot be absorbed into the hairs and the results may be disappointing.

The best way to resolve the problem is to use an eyelash dye on the affected hairs. This procedure needs to be repeated every six weeks or so as the hairs grow out and are replaced by new ones. While this can be done professionally in a beauty salon, many patients, particularly men and boys, prefer to do it for themselves to save personal embarrassment.

You must explain the correct procedure for eyelash dyeing to the patient. If the brows are also affected and need treatment, you must warn that the dye takes very quickly on brows and will need to be removed before the eyelash dyeing is completed.

9

Care of the skin

The skin consists of three layers: the deepest level is the subcutaneous layer, the central layer is the dermis, or true skin, and the outer layer is the epidermis.

The subcutaneous or fatty layer serves as a buffer to the underlying structures of the body; its thickness differs in different people, between men and women, and also varies from one area of the body to another. It is this layer of the skin which acts as an insulator against heat and cold, and provides the body contours. Dieting – or controlled intake of calories – is based on the assumption that, if the intake of food is less than that needed for the energy output, the body consumes some of the subcutaneous layer and this slims the shape. The problem is that the fat used is not necessarily from the particular parts where slimness is desired.

The middle layer, the dermis, is the most important of the three layers of the skin. It is a fibrous mass of tissue which includes fibres of elastin and collagen, and is referred to as connective tissue, because it links the two other layers. The cells of the dermis all contain a nucleus and are therefore alive. New cells are formed in the basal layer of the dermis to replace those which have worked their way up to the outer surface of the skin and been shed. The dermis is fed by the blood capillaries it contains. Also within the dermis are the nerve endings – through which we recognise heat, cold, touch and pain – the sweat glands which regulate the temperature of the skin as well as secreting certain waste products, and hair roots with their attached sebaceous glands. Lastly, the dermis contains cells which manufacture melanin, the substance which determines our skin colour and allows the skin to tan when exposed to sunlight.

The epidermis is sometimes referred to as the horny layer. As the dermal cells pass into this top layer they become flattened, lose their nucleii and die, and thus form the hard surface, which is the body's first defence against infection and foreign bodies. As new cells are taken in from the basal layer on the underside of the

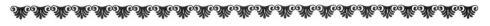

epidermis, the cells in the top layer of the epidermis detach themselves, having completed their life cycle.

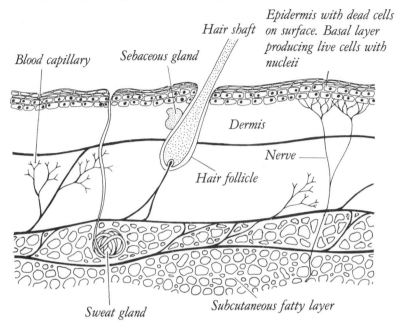

Blood capillary   *Sebaceous gland*   *Hair shaft*   *Epidermis with dead cells on surface. Basal layer producing live cells with nucleii*

Dermis

Nerve

Hair follicle

Sweat gland   *Subcutaneous fatty layer*

The skin is waterproof, being a one-way system for the outward passage of liquids. When bathing, the crinkling effect you get on the skin after being too long in water, noticeable particularly on the fingers, is caused by loss of water from within the body. If water is placed on the skin, it can only evaporate. In doing this it uses up natural body heat and at the same time allows some of the natural moisture to escape from the skin.

Therefore, it is not difficult to see that when water is used to wash the face, it merely cleans away surface dirt. Soap is alkaline, whereas the natural oily protection on the skin is acidic. When an alkali is added to an acid the two are neutralised, so the use of soap and water together removes surface dirt as well as the natural fats present for the protection of the skin, leaving the skin temporarily unprotected.

What soap and water cannot do is penetrate the skin to extract the dirt trapped in the pores. The 'clean' feeling associated with a soap and water face wash is caused by the removal of the natural fats which leaves the skin feeling taut, and this sensation has quite erroneously been associated with cleanliness.

Skin tends to be categorised as normal, dry, oily, or a combination of these, but these are not good definitions. A child before puberty could be said to have a normal skin. At this stage of development the skin is fine, smooth and evenly textured as well as being elastic and soft, but after puberty many changes occur. The increased hormonal activity during puberty can cause an imbalance of glandular secretions, perhaps leading to an over-production of sebum by the sebaceous glands, which in turn can lead to the distressing condition, acne. Hormones also cause the male skin to thicken at puberty and the female skin to reduce in thickness.

After reaching puberty, skin can tend either to dryness – sometimes in patches, or to greasiness – again not always all over the skin. Some faces tend to have an oily area in the centre, which results in blocked pores, leading to spots mainly around the forehead, nose and chin while the cheeks are dry.

Consider the patient who suffers an over-production of sebum, the substance produced in the sebaceous glands attached to the hair follicles. Because hair is mainly above the face, the sebum drops from the hair on to the face, clogging the pores and causing spots. When this happens many people style their hair to try to cover up the spots. This creates a vicious circle in which more sebum is deposited on the face to cause more spots. Most people suffering from this problem then feel that as their skin must be oily, putting more oil on the skin is the wrong thing to do. However, the opposite is true. The oil is able to penetrate the outer layer of the skin by mixing naturally with the protective fats on the skin. Thus if oil is used as a cleanser it helps to stabilise any excess secretion, and leaves the skin clean without removing completely the protective layer of fats.

Dry skins have a different problem in that they become prone to wrinkles through a lack of moisture. One cause of dryness can be exposure to the ultra-violet rays in sunlight. This affects all types of skin but shows more quickly in the dry-skinned patient. Heredity plays a part in your skin type and it is often said – if you want to know what a girl will look like later in life, look at her mother. While there is some truth in this saying, remember that people also inherit from their fathers.

No matter what type of skin you have, the important thing is to be sure to cleanse it thoroughly and that means more than just the top surface. You must make sure that whatever cleansing agent you use, it penetrates into the pores and stops dirt being trapped below the epidermis. To do this the cleansing agent must contain a higher percentage of oil than water.

Unfortunately, manufacturers of cosmetics seldom list the contents of their products, apparently considering the packaging and presentation more important than the contents. The cosmetics industry – like any other – is in the business for profit, and wishes to persuade the public that its products will be beneficial and will add glamour and lustre to the appearance. The public condones this view by accepting that the manufacturer's name is all that matters and that if a product is highly priced it must do more good than a cheaper brand. This is rarely true.

Basically all creams contain both oil and water. Those which have a higher percentage of water than of oil are known as oil-in-water emulsions, while those containing a higher percentage of oil than of water are known as water-in-oil emulsions. The thinner the consistency, the more likely the product is to be an oil-in-water emulsion. Remembering that the higher the water content, the cheaper the cream should be to produce, it is not surprising that many creams and lotions fall into the oil-in-water category. As the water in the cream cannot have any beneficial effect on the skin, the oil-in-water products can do very little good. Indeed water causes dryness – for with evaporation of the water in the cream some of the skin's natural moisture content will also escape.

Many cleansing milks are oil-in-water emulsions and therefore cannot clean the skin efficiently. Tonics and toners are almost completely water and for the same reason also dry the skin, being incapable of penetrating it. Some tonics also contain alcohol and this can do positive harm.

Moisturisers are sometimes claimed to put moisture (water) into the skin but it is known that this is impossible because the skin is waterproof. Many moisturisers come into the category of oil-in-water products, containing only small quantities of oil. Until the type and proportion of contents are clearly listed on product labels, it will be impossible to know which contain water-in-oil emulsions which are beneficial to the skin.

All these facts tend to make your choice difficult. Standard manufacturers' literature says we should cleanse our faces and then use a toner or astringent to close the pores before applying a moisturiser. However, you can see that if soap and water or an oil-in-water emulsion is used for cleansing, all you achieve is the removal of the skin's natural moisture. This is an expensive and time-consuming exercise for doing nothing but harm, and the skin pores remain clogged with dirt.

Therefore, when choosing a cleansing cream, it is important to enquire what basic type of emulsion it is even though sales assistants are often reluctant to tell you and may not know themselves. To be of benefit to the skin, the cleanser must be a water-in-oil emulsion.

There is a simple answer, you can make your own. At least then you will know what you are putting on your face. Here is an easy recipe to follow, and the whole process will take you under half an hour.

Ingredients for cleansing cream

	Imperial	Metric	American
Beeswax	1 oz	28 g	1 oz
Liquid paraffin	7 fl oz	200 ml	1 cup – scant ½ pint
Borax	⅓ level teaspoonful	⅓ of a 5 ml spoon	⅓ level teaspoonful
Boiling water	5 fl oz/¼ pint	142 ml	⅔ cup

Note Beeswax, which can be yellow or white, is obtainable at some chemists, health food stores, art and craft shops and some hardware stores. Liquid paraffin and borax can be bought in chemists shops.

Method

1) Place the beeswax and liquid paraffin together in a basin (glass or china) over a saucepan of boiling water (NOT DIRECT HEAT) and leave until the beeswax has melted. (Approximately 10 min.) Remove from heat.
2) At this point and in a separate receptacle pour the boiling water over the borax. Stir well but do not use a mixer.
3) Add the borax and water solution to the beeswax and liquid paraffin solution, stir well by hand and pour into small clean pots to cool.

If you pour out the mix while it is still hot the basin will be easy to clean but if you wait until the cream has set (3 to 4 hours) the basin will be very greasy and difficult to clean. The quantities stated will produce approximately one pound of cream.

From the quantities of ingredients used you will see that this produces a water-in-oil emulsion. As explained, this is the only type of emulsion which can have a beneficial effect on the skin.

First apply cleansing cream all over the face, making sure that every part has been covered. Secondly remove all this cream with a piece of damp cotton wool which can then be thrown away. All traces of cream must be removed from the skin and this method of cleansing should be used both night and morning instead of soap and water. It is the correct and efficient way to clean the skin.

When you start to use this method of cleansing, particularly if you previously used soap and water, spots may appear, showing that there was dirt to be extracted from the pores. If you cleanse the skin correctly with cream for a period of 7 to 10 days no more spots should appear, the skin by now being thoroughly clean. At the end of a 2-week period of correct cleansing the skin will be softer and smoother, with previously blocked enlarged pores beginning to diminish in size.

Even though moisture cannot penetrate the skin, a very fine film of water-in-oil emulsion applied all over the face can trap the skin's own moisture inside. This is the real function of a moisturiser. The cleansing cream described above, being a water-in-oil emulsion, is an ideal all purpose cream on all types of skin and can therefore be used for cleansing and as a moisturiser to trap the skin's natural moisture.

A knowledge of proper skin care is the key to success in cosmetic camouflage. Often scars will be presented with poor skin condition around them. The application of cover creams will be inhibited and the effect spoiled by a spotty or erupting surrounding skin and it is important that you explain to the patient that an improvement can be made, and that this will give a much better result to the camouflage. Indeed, the scars themselves can become softer and more pliable with proper deep cleansing.

For those who have always used a liquid make-up base on their faces, remember that these, too, are basically water with colouring matter added. They will therefore cause the skin's natural moisture to evaporate as they dry. The colouring matter can also clog the pores, the first step in the formation of spots.

Most people who use foundation creams do so out of habit, thinking that imperfections will be hidden – while in fact these creams may be the cause of future problems, especially after continual use. However, if you can establish the correct cleansing procedure and you find the skin softer and healthier after only 2 weeks, perhaps you will be prepared to embark on a completely new make-up routine, which carries on the principle of using only water-in-oil products.

If you use a little skin-matching cover cream, not over the whole of the face, but to hide any imperfections, you will not need a liquid make-up base. The technique is first to apply a very thin film of water-in-oil emulsion as a moisturiser, then use the cover cream to hide any imperfections, and finally cover the face liberally with a translucent powder, brushing off the excess with dry cotton wool. Eyeshadow and blusher can then be added as necessary. If a damp cotton wool swab is pressed gently all over the face at this stage the matt look will last longer.

Instead of applying more powder during the day to hide any perspiration you can blot the face carefully with a damp cotton wool swab. This way the make-up stays matt with no additions. Thus it is a good idea to carry several damp cotton wool swabs with you in a small plastic bag.

A liquid make-up base can be useful however on one part of the face –surprisingly, the lips. If you apply a little to the lips and powder before using a lip pencil to outline the shape, you can then fill in the outline with lipstick using a small brush, and you get a clearly defined mouth which will remain stable for most of the day.

If you use the correct procedure for cleansing over several weeks and some whiteheads and blackheads persist there is a simple routine you can try. This consists of mixing a little oil with some ordinary oatmeal and very gently rubbing this into the spotty area. The mixture acts as a mild abrasive which should remove the troublesome spots near the surface. The routine should not be done more than once each week and you must also remember never to remove, or try to remove spots by pressing them with the fingers, because you will cause further inflammation and probably more spots to appear alongside. Surface veins can also be damaged if you press too hard.

Night creams can be of some benefit because these creams are most likely to be water-in-oil products. However, after cleansing the skin properly at night, unless it is very dry, you would be sensible to allow it to breathe uncluttered by anything when it needs no protection from wind, rain and dirt. In the case of very dry or elderly skins a thin film of water-in-oil emulsion would help to retain natural moisture during the night.

10

Prosthetics

For the clinical cosmetician to play her full part in the rehabilitation of the patient, it is essential that she knows and understands the various techniques which may be used to improve the quality of the patient's life. Nowadays it is not enough merely to save life but steps must be taken to provide the patient with a fully acceptable appearance in society so that life may be enjoyed to the full.

A great deal of progress has been made in this field since the days when, for instance, leg amputees would have been supplied with wooden stumps to enable them to walk. At that time they would have been expected to live with the pain and discomfort and no thought would have been given to their appearance, or to the effect it would have on their life-style.

We now have some understanding of the mental anxiety and stress that can be caused by the loss of a limb or any bodily disfigurement. From an awareness of how the mind and spirit of the patient can be affected, new ideas have developed of the various aspects of healing which need to be considered. Cosmetic camouflage is one of these, and I hope it will become a readily available service with a large number of dedicated people to do it. Another essential service that has emerged in the past few decades is prosthetics.

A prosthesis is any manufactured appendage used to complete or complement the human body. It is an artificial part made to rectify a defect and the name derives from a Greek word meaning 'to replace'. Even false nails, teeth or eyelashes can be termed prostheses. In the wider sense prostheses include artificial limbs, eyes, ears and any part of the anatomy which can be manufactured to simulate living tissue.

The art of making prostheses to hide disfigurement has been practised for thousands of years, as we know from archeologists who have discovered false ears, noses and eyes fashioned in a variety of materials including porcelain, silver and gold, from the Egyptian period of about 2500 BC. Egyptologists suggest that these prostheses were probably made after death, so that the wearers would be more presentable to meet their gods. Although delicately fashioned, most of them were cumbersome and heavy. They would not, therefore, have been made as an aid to rehabilitation and were probably made by the mortician.

Any prostheses made prior to the Egyptian period would have been of clay or animal skins, and would not have had the durability to survive for us to see.

Today there are many more materials and substances available for reconstructive work by technicians including rubber, plastic, acrylics and silicone, and the search goes on for the perfect medium.

The technicians who construct facial prostheses are dedicated people who have qualified as dental technicians and then studied the subject of facial prosthetics over a number of years. They are known as maxillo-facial technicians and their skills and inventiveness enable them to work closely with the surgeons on complicated cases requiring reconstruction of both boney areas and the skin.

Where deformity occurs inside the mouth (intra orally), it can cause speech problems as well as an inability to control food and liquid. Where reconstruction is not possible with surgery, technicians can often devise something to help the patient eat, drink and communicate.

Unfortunately not all hospitals can offer the services of these technicians and if they are not available, patients have to be referred elsewhere. The ideal situation allows the technician to work closely with the surgeon, with continuing discussion of the most suitable solution to the patient's problem.

It may be that all the defects presented by the patient can eventually be resolved by surgery, with the grafting of both bone and skin, but these procedures are carried out step by step over a considerable period of time. The natural healing process is slow and cannot be hurried, necessitating delays between operations, yet the patient must still be able to meet friends and relations in the interim periods. In such cases it may be possible to construct a temporary prosthesis that will hide the affected parts of the face. Loss of the nose would be such a case. Because the nose is so important to the look of the face, the waiting period before the start of surgery would be a difficult time for the patient, and a temporary prosthesis attached to a spectacles frame could be a great help.

The ear is a particularly difficult area for a surgeon to reconstruct. A prosthetic ear attached by adhesive not only looks completely natural but is easy to wear. Where there is little left of the natural ear, it can be advisable to remove the small area of remaining ear tissue to give a good flat surface for the prosthetic ear, rather than attempting reconstruction. The prosthesis will have been matched exactly in colour and shape to the patient's existing ear and will sharpen and focus sound to the inner ear in exactly the same way as the natural ear. For a deaf patient it would be possible to fix a deaf aid inside the prosthesis, thus improving the quality of the patient's life as well as his or her appearance.

Where patients have undergone surgery for the removal of a tumour, it may not be possible to use grafts for reconstruction. When this applies to the cheeks or the eye and its orbit, a prosthesis which has been moulded exactly to fit the remaining contours of the face can be attached to the patient's spectacles. Although the weight of the prosthesis is less than that of the diseased tissue which has been removed, it can sit heavily on the bridge of the nose causing redness. In this case it might be necessary to camouflage the problem area. Normally such prostheses are made of rigid material which must withstand the possibility of fading in sunlight and constant cleaning to remove the effects of smoke and dirt in the atmosphere, and yet be fine enough to look natural. Very recently a real breakthrough has been made in the manufacture of prostheses. It has been found possible to produce a prosthesis for one side of the face, including the orbit, which extends on to the forehead and is attached by a new special adhesive. It does not need to be attached to spectacles and therefore can be worn without removal for days or even weeks at a time. It so closely resembles living tissue that the appearance is remarkably normal. Sometimes a problem occurs when the surrounding skin changes colour with the seasons; as a cosmetician you may be asked to use camouflage on the prosthesis to match this change in colour.

You should be aware of the possibility that a patient who wears a facial prosthesis may then remove it to reveal the absence of part of the face. Hot weather can cause chafing at the edge of a prosthesis and you may be called upon to camouflage the inflamed area. You will find that a number of patients will have facial prostheses which are not apparent at first glance. A prosthetic eye which fits perfectly into a patients' orbit, and is beautifully matched with the existing eye, will be particularly difficult to recognise, especially where muscle action has been maintained to give natural movement.

Breast augmentation is another situation which concerns the cosmetician. This may have been carried out for aesthetic reasons, where lack of shape caused the patient concern, or for the patient who has undergone mastectomy (removal of the breast). A prosthesis can either be made to simulate the whole breast, or placed as an implant under the remaining tissue to match the contour on the other side. As a cosmetician you may be required to camouflage the scarring left from these operations. For your information, the implants are small round cushions of transparent material filled with a colourless fluid.

Where a nipple has been removed during mastectomy, a plastic surgeon can sometimes fashion a replacement with a graft. However, it is worth noting that plastic nipples are available in the United Kingdom from the manufacturers, Strodex Ltd, Strodex House, Nottingham Road, Long Eaton NG10 1JW (tel. 060 76 2203). While reconstructed nipples are preferable, in cases where this is impossible a soft plastic replacement can be an acceptable alternative for a mutilated patient.

HAIR

The area of prosthetics of particular importance to the cosmetician is hair. You should be thoroughly familiar with all aspects of hair, including eyelashes and brows, as well as wigs.

Wigs

Wigs are normally ordered from and fitted by a reputable wig-maker, and this is not your concern, but you may well see patients who have to wear a wig following the loss of their own hair and who are having difficulty with either the maintenance of the wig or the method of attaching it securely.

A wig (or postiche) made by a wig-maker from real hair has had each strand individually knotted on to the foundation vegetable netting on the circumference and the looser woven caul net of the crown. As with natural hair, wigs and postiches need to be set after cleaning and must therefore be taken to a hairdresser who provides this service.

Less expensive than a real hair wig is one made of synthetic fibre. The fibres are woven on to a cap foundation and as the caps are not individually fitted they can be altered in size by the use of stretch elastic in the nape. After washing, artificial wigs do not need re-setting and can be brushed into the required style quite easily.

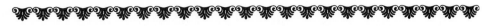

Washing should be done frequently so that the base is kept free from sweat which could cause rotting.

A full wig of human hair is made exactly to fit the wearer and should pose no problem in wear. Part pieces, however, will need to be secured either by the small combs attached to them, or by postiche clips. Where a small amount of natural hair still remains on the scalp, it can be used as a base for securing a wig or hairpiece. This is done in the following way:

Take a few strands of the natural hair and roll them into a small curl (a) securing with a hair grip (b). Place a second grip on the curl, at right angles to the first (c). Repeat wherever enough natural hair is available. Then place the wig or hairpiece in position over the grips which can be felt through it. Take a fine hairpin, slip it through the wig into the cross made by the two grips and push it downwards to sit close to the scalp. The hairpiece will now be firm and can be brushed into the required style.

(a)   (b)   (c)

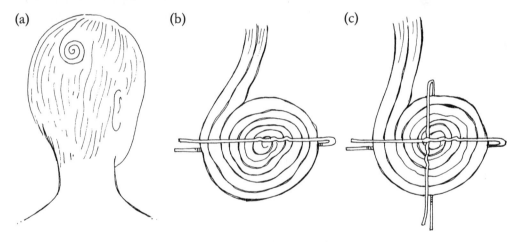

A wig which has been individually produced for a patient by the wig-maker will have been fashioned to give a natural effect around the face. This does not apply to wigs made of synthetic fibres, which all too often are spoiled by a hard line where they meet the face.

When a fashion wig is purchased it should be chosen to match as nearly as possible the colour of the natural hair. Thus when the wig is in place, wisps of the natural hair can be pulled out and combed or brushed into the wig to give a natural hairline. This not only improves the appearance but gives the wig added stability. A toupee wearer can buy double-sided adhesive tape to attach the hairpiece firmly to the scalp.

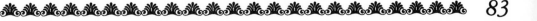

Eyebrows

Facial burns or other trauma can cause the loss of eyebrows and this is a problem which can worry patients. The use of eyebrow pencils is covered in Chapter 6, *Methods of Application,* but this does not always give a satisfactory result, particularly with men. Where hair is available from other parts of the body, a plastic surgeon can apply a hair-bearing graft to form new brows and these will need to be trimmed from time to time to maintain a natural appearance. Grafts of this type are also used to disguise loss of contour of the upper lip by forming a moustache, or on the jaw as a beard.

Where no natural body hair is available, the maxillo-facial technician is able to make an eyebrow based on a slim strip of plastic which is attached by adhesive over the brow bone, giving a good natural effect.

Another solution is to use crepe hair, of the type used by actors and actresses. Crepe hair is relatively cheap and is available from theatrical costumiers, being sold by the metre in five or six different shades. To give a natural effect, you should tease several shades together – take strands from the plaited lengths and roll them together between your fingers. If both brows are missing, then you should prepare enough for two eyebrows at the same time to be sure of an exact match. The new brows should be trimmed to the approximate size of a natural brow and pressed firmly on to the brow bone which has already been spread with adhesive, usually spirit gum. Apply firm pressure for a few seconds until the attachment is secure and then trim the brows into shape with small sharp scissors.

This method produces a bushy type of brow which looks particularly natural on men. With female patients, smaller eyebrows give a better appearance and these can be made in exactly the same way – but before teasing the colours together you must straighten the crepe hair, by pulling it taut while passing it quickly through the steam from a boiling kettle. Smaller and neater brows can be made with straight hair. Crepe brows need to be replaced frequently and therefore this type of substitute brow should only be considered as a last resort, when no other method is possible.

Eyelashes

A lack of definition in the face can be caused by the permanent loss of eyelashes through trauma. Not only is the appearance affected; eyelashes act as a natural shade for the eyes and without them the eyes can water a lot in strong light causing inflammation and embarrassment.

It is possible for lashes to be grafted on to the lids by a plastic surgeon. There is, however, a risk that the lashes in the graft may not grow, and as the life of a lash is only about six weeks, this difficult and often painful procedure might also be pointless. Thus very few of these grafts are undertaken.

False eyelashes

There are two main types of false eyelashes. First is the type manufactured as individual lashes, to be used in addition to remaining natural lashes (a). Each lash consists of several fine hairs fixed into a tiny root (b). This root is attached with adhesive to the base of the natural existing lash – not to the eyelid – so that when several are attached in this way along the length of the lid the effect is very natural (c).

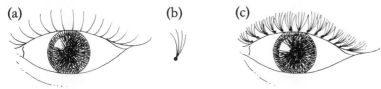

These eyelashes are waterproof and when correctly attached will stay in place for a considerable time. However they cannot last longer than the lash to which they are attached.

The second type of manufactured lashes is made as a set, to be secured along the edge of the eyelid with special adhesives. These lashes are manufactured in various thicknesses, the finest usually being recommended for daytime use. Daytime fine eyelashes are the most suitable for a natural appearance and for permanent wear. Before you apply them, you must trim them to the correct size for the patient.

First you must measure the width of the eye. False lashes are produced in the largest possible widths, so almost always you will need to cut away a little to match the width of the patient's eye This should always be done at the end where the lashes are longest, that is, the outside (a).

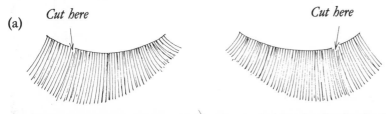

Natural lashes are all different lengths according to the stage of their growth, so the false lashes should be trimmed to match. This is done in the following way (b): use small sharp scissors to clip into, and not across, the lashes all the way along until they are uneven.

(b)
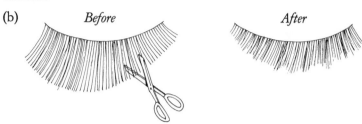
Before　　　　　　　　　　　*After*

Attaching false lashes

Points to remember

1) For small eyes it is better to buy half-lashes or three-quarter lashes.
2) False lashes are never attached right into the inner corner of the eye, but to about 5 mm from it.
3) If the patient has an allergy to the normal adhesive, you must obtain the special adhesives that some cosmetic manufacturers produce.
4) Remove false lashes by holding the outside and gently peeling off towards the nose, thus eliminating the possibility of dragging the lid.

Top lashes

Before preparing the false lashes make sure the eyelids are free from grease and dirt.

1) Apply adhesive along the straight edge of the false lashes. This can be done in either of two ways:
    (a) Place a small amount of adhesive in the palm of the hand and transfer it to the false lashes with the pointed end of an orange stick.
    (b) Apply directly from the tube of adhesive onto the false lashes – but take care!
2) Using the blunt end of the orange stick, now press the centre of the lashes down on to the centre of the eyelid, as close to the natural lashes as possible. Press the lashes down working along the lid, first to the left and then to the right.
3) Remove any excess adhesive before it has set, because after setting it will be colourless and difficult to see. If any excess is left on the skin, it will feel tacky and may spoil the make-up applied later.

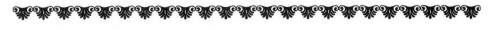

4) With a mascara brush, blend together the natural lashes with the false ones.
5) Using an eyeliner, fill in any gaps on the edge of the lids.
6) Apply mascara, if absolutely necessary, first by brushing it along the top of the lashes, then finishing with a lifting movement from underneath.

Lower lashes

It is rarely necessary to apply lower lashes, because the resulting effect can be rather heavy. However, younger patients may request it. You can use the same procedure as for the upper lashes, except that when you apply the lashes the patient must look upwards, and the false lashes must be placed underneath the natural lashes.

It is possible, though more difficult, to apply false lashes where no natural ones exist. In this case you must take great care to attach the false lashes as close to the edge of the eyelid as possible, and in addition you will need to apply an eyeliner to give definition to the edge of the lid.

In some situations, an eyeliner can be a good solution by itself, and this is explained in Chapter 6, *Methods of Application,* under highlighting and shading. The use of false lashes where no natural lashes exist is not recommended for either male or elderly patients.

Care of false lashes

False lashes can be re-used many times but old adhesive must be removed after each wearing. For this simply use warm soapy water.

The eyelashes should be placed on a tissue or cloth and tapped sharply, several times, using a toothbrush loaded with warm soapy water. This should loosen the dirt and adhesive, which can then be peeled off with tweezers.

Curling false eyelashes

False lashes have a much better appearance when they have been curled and this is a simple procedure. (See following page.)
1) Clean the lashes as described above.
2) Take a paper tissue and a round pencil (a).
3) Lay the cleaned top lashes the right way up on the tissue, at one end of its length (b).
4) Place the pencil on top of the lashes (c).
5) Now roll the tissue tightly – starting at the pencil end – using the palms of the hands and the fingers to do this, so

that the lashes and the pencil are contained in the rolled-up tissue (d).

6) Put an elastic band round each end of the rolled tissue (e).
7) Leave for several hours or overnight. The lashes will then be dry, have a gentle curl, and be ready for reapplication.

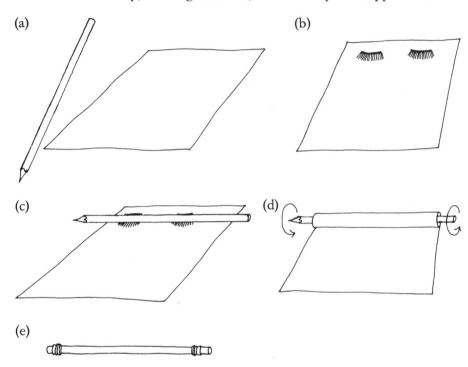

(a)

(b)

(c)

(d)

(e)

An alternative method, which curls the lashes permanently, is to paint them with clear lacquer after cleaning and use greaseproof paper to roll them rather than a tissue.

In conclusion, it must be stated that for cosmetic camouflage you need to be inventive, but in some cases you may still find it impossible to produce a result that is fully satisfactory, either to yourself or to the patient. In such cases, you might want to contact a maxillo-facial technician about the possibility of a prosthesis being constructed. It is wise therefore to make contact with a technician and try to establish a rapport *before* you need help. You can then find out in which particular field he or she excels and check the correct procedure for requesting help. This can be of mutual benefit as the technician may be glad to know of your work and may find it helpful to be able to refer patients to you. Approached

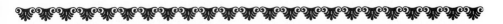

in the right way these dedicated technicians are usually prepared to make a prosthesis even for such unusual requests as filling a hole in a leg, or fashioning a nipple lost due to mastectomy – neither of which conditions can be helped with the application of cover cream!

11

Medical terminology

Today, as in the past, the medical profession in general casts a sceptical eye on the beauty profession and its sometimes exaggerated claims for the treatments it offers. Perhaps the clinical cosmetician will be able – with her knowledge of cosmetic camouflage – to bridge the gap which exists at present, given that there are already areas of health care in which both professions hold the same viewpoint. One example is the problem of excess weight, a condition so damaging to health. New establishments are constantly being opened to cater for the increasing demand for healthy exercise and the beauty profession provides attractive venues which give encouragement and support to their clients.

Beauty establishments are well supported by the public, with many clients constantly searching for new products and treatments which they hope may achieve the impossible. In the field of electrolysis the beautician's work is invaluable and massage can relieve tension and promote a feeling of well being, so that a client's appearance must be improved.

As a clinical cosmetician, however, you must consider your role as a para-medical one. If you are fortunate enough to work in a hospital you will be part of a team and will need a vocabulary that allows you to participate fully in discussions regarding patient welfare.

While no one will expect you to have a complete knowledge of medicine, you should be able to understand at least where the problems are sited and what, if anything, is possible with medical or surgical treatment. This knowledge will not only lead you to a deeper involvement with your work but also bring you greater satisfaction and make you a more respected member of the medical team. You will also need to understand the medical terminology used in letters of referral from consultants or general practitioners about their patients.

Some of your referrals will undoubtedly come from consultant plastic surgeons. This work covers a wide field but can be summarised under six main headings:

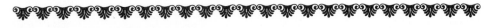

1) treatment of burns and scars
2) congenital abnormalities
3) hand injuries and abnormalities
4) treatment of facial trauma
5) head and neck cancer
6) cosmetic surgery

The word 'plastic' derives from the Greek 'plastikos' meaning 'having the power to give form, capable of being moulded or modelled, forming living tissue'. Therefore the plastic surgeon moulds living tissue and this use of the word is not in any way concerned with the current popular understanding of plastics. (In the United Kingdom a plastic surgeon holds a postgraduate surgical qualification as well as a medical degree, so he or she should be addressed as Mr (or equivalent) and not Doctor.)

The para-medical team assisting a plastic surgeon is likely to include a physiotherapist, who uses massage, manipulation and other techniques to restore function to limbs, an occupational therapist, who assists in the rehabilitation of the patient, and a clinical cosmetician who may be able to help patients for whom surgery is unsuitable and will also be able to improve the appearance of those who have undergone surgery. Another specialist who will attend clinics from time to time will be the maxillo-facial consultant, who will be consulted about facial bone grafting, teeth and so on. Finally, there will probably be a psychiatrist, whose guidance may be sought on the patient's suitability for a particular type of treatment.

Much of a plastic surgeon's work will involve skin grafting, which may in discussion be referred to as 'flaps'. Thus when patients are mentioned as having 'flaps', this is not a reference to their mental states but instead that they are undergoing a type of skin grafting! A 'flap' is defined as a tongue or lip of tissue cut away from the underlying parts but left attached at one end for its blood supply. It is used in plastic surgery for filling a defect in a neighbouring region, or to cover the cut end of the bone after amputation.

GRAFTS

A skin graft is a layer of skin cut from one area (the donor site) and transferred to a new site. Depending on the nature of the site where the graft is to be laid, it will be thin, thick or a split thickness of skin. A general rule is that the thinner the graft, the more easily it will be accepted on the recipient site, but the appearance will not be as good as with a full thickness of skin, which would give the best result for colour, texture and movement. Recently advances in microsurgical vascular techniques, using special microscopes, have made it possible to transpose a piece of skin with its muscles, tissues and blood vessels intact.

Grafts are used for a number of reasons:

1) to replace dead tissue after burning
2) to close an area which will not heal normally
3) to provide skin with which to fashion a replacement feature, such as a nose, tongue or eyelid
4) to provide covering where the original tissue has had to be removed.

Because a graft is acceptable only if taken from the patient's own body, there has to be enough suitable healthy skin available.

In the case of a split thickness or thin graft – usually taken from the thigh – ten days must elapse before the graft can be said to have 'taken', during which time it is essential that there be little or no movement of the affected part. For this type of graft, more skin than would appear to be necessary is taken from the donor site; the excess is kept under refrigeration and can be preserved for up to twenty one days, so that if the original graft has not taken at the end of ten days, another can be applied from the preserved spare skin. Even a third graft is possible, on the twenty first day. After the skin to be grafted has been removed from the donor site, this resembles a very bad graze so it is kept covered and undisturbed so that new skin will form naturally. The cover or bandage on the donor site will be left to fall off naturally, about the twenty first day, when a new skin will have been formed. It is worth noting that little or no pain will be felt at the site of the graft but the donor site will be painful mainly due to contact with the thick bandages.

A **flap** is a full thickness area of tissue that is left temporarily attached to the donor site and to its blood supply.

A **direct flap** is one which is sutured to the defect.

An **island flap,** or tube pedicle, is a double-ended tubed stalk of skin and subcutaneous tissue containing a blood supply, which is moved in stages from one site to another – a procedure taking some weeks. When the blood supply has been established at the new site, the graft is detached from its original site and secured completely on to its new siting. By this means a graft can be removed from the forearm to, say, the forehead, the arm being securely fastened to the forehead for the whole period and the blood supply being maintained throughout. This technique is used

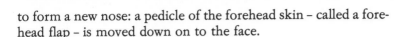

to form a new nose: a pedicle of the forehead skin – called a fore-head flap – is moved down on to the face.

A delayed flap is one for which reattachment is postponed until after elimination of infection and formation of a bed of healthy granulation tissue on the new site.

A hair-bearing graft is taken from a donor area of hair-bearing skin – such as the scalp — in order to replace eyebrows, or to form a beard or moustache to mask a deformity.

KELOID SCARS

Put simply, keloid scars can often look like rotted elastic and are usually raised and discoloured. They are fairly common and occur more frequently in Negroid skins. The cause of this condition is not yet known but it is most likely to occur on earlobes, chin, neck, shoulders and upper trunk (the so-called cape area).

It can occur in the dermis and adjacent subcutaneous tissue, usually after trauma, burns, surgery or vaccination. It frequently recurs in the skin after surgical removal.

The medical definition is 'a nodular, frequently lobulated, unusually firm, moveable, non-encapsulated, generally linear mass of peculiar hyperplastic scar tissue consisting of relatively large and fairly parallel bands of densely collagenous material separated by bands of cellular fibrous tissue'.

Plastic surgeons are loath to remove such scars surgically, par-ticularly where the surrounding skin is taut with no looseness of tissue around the scar, as a larger keloid would probably be formed. There are several methods of dealing with this condition that can bring considerable improvement and even eradication.

1) intralesional steroid injections
2) wearing a specially fitted pressure garment, such as a Jobst garment
3) application of a steroid impregnated sticky tape, for example Haelan tape
4) deep X-ray therapy

These methods require considerable time to take effect but the final results can fully justify their application. Different surgeons tend to favour one method rather than another.

'W' AND 'Z' PLASTY

Ordinary scars can be removed surgically, leaving neater and less obvious scars in their place which can probably be completely hidden by camouflage. Sometimes an improvement can be made to a scar by means of a technique known as 'W' and 'Z' plasty.

This procedure is used particularly where a scar or lesion has grown taut and is causing a slight bulging effect in the surrounding tissue: in the face the features can be distorted. The scar can be 'eased' by cutting it in the line of relaxed skin tension – as the name suggests – in the shape of a continuous W or Z. This can be more clearly understood by comparing it to a dressmaking technique: where tension can cause splitting in a garment, the fabric needs to be cut on the cross. Again in dressmaking, a strategically placed insert or dart which will not split with movement, allows the fabric to fall naturally and softly.

There are a great number of procedures undertaken by plastic surgeons and it is useful for you to know the names of the ones most likely to be used for patients who will be referred to you.

A face lift refers to the whole face.

Blepharoplasty means any operation for the restoration of a defect on the eyelids and can be called a partial face lift.

Rhinoplasty means any restorative or reconstructive plastic surgery to the nose; it can be the supplying of a partial or complete replacement of the nose, by tissue taken from elsewhere.

Dermabrasion is the operative procedure mainly used for the reduction of acne scarring. It may be performed using sand-paper, wire brushes or other abrasive materials.

Breast augmentation is the surgical procedure for the implanting of prostheses in the breasts in order to give shape and fullness.

Breast reduction is the removal of some of the excess subcutaneous layer in the breasts, together with the associated excess skin.

Note Where a mastectomy has involved the complete removal of the breast including the nipple, a plastic surgeon can reform a nipple by grafting to give a near-normal appearance to the breast.

These are mainly cosmetic surgery procedures, and form only a small part of most plastic surgeons' work, with reconstructive surgery to the face, neck and hands being commonplace. Never-

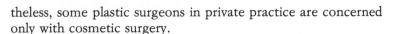

theless, some plastic surgeons in private practice are concerned only with cosmetic surgery.

To add to the list of conditions which you could meet as a cosmetician on the plastic surgery unit, here is a list of conditions and medical terms with which you should become familiar.

Biopsy is the process of removing tissue from living patients for diagnostic examination.

Carcinoma is a malignant growth.

Contact allergy is an abnormal sensitivity to a substance (allergen or antigen), which results in an unwanted and excessive inflammatory reaction. There are several types of allergic response; the form the clinical cosmetician is most likely to come across is contact allergic dermatitis (contact eczema), which is a form of cell mediated delayed allergy. Common causes of contact allergic dermatitis are perfumes, lanolin, topical antibiotics, colophony in Elastoplast and nickel in watches and costume jewellery. Not all dermatitis is due to allergy.

Contact irritant dermatitis is far more common than contact allergy and is due to direct physical and chemical damage to the skin, for example from soap, water, wind, detergents, oil, grease and tar. Some forms of dermatitis occur as a result of hereditary or endogenous factors (originating from within), for example atopic dermatitis (infantile eczema).

Haematoma is a collection of blood under the skin.

Hypertrophy is a general increase in bulk of part of an organ, not due to tumour formation.

Jobst garment is an elasticated garment which conforms to the shape of the body to exert pressure; it is custom made to fit the individual patient and is used extensively for burns scars to prevent contracture and to restore flatness and smoothness and normal colour to the healing tissue.

Lesion is a general term for injury, swelling or abnormality.

Lipoma is a benign tumour of fat, i.e. one which is not malignant.

Melanin is the pigmented substance in the dermis which gives the skin its colour. It is produced by melanocytes.

Melanocytic naevus or mole is a birthmark containing melanin and is relatively common. On occasions these may change their character, developing abnormalities in later life and when this happens, camouflage should be avoided until medical advice is taken. Great care should be taken not to remove any hairs present, either by shaving or other means, without taking medical advice.

Nodules can be seen and felt on the skin and may involve the full depth of skin.

Oncology is the science, study and care of tumours.

Orbit is an eye socket.

Pigmentation is the colouring produced by melanin.
> *Hypopigmentation* – loss of colour compared with the surrounding skin.
> *Hyperpigmentation* – excess of colour compared with the surrounding skin.

Prognosis is an opinion as to the probable result of an illness.

Rodent ulcer is a locally malignant ulcerating tumour, occurring mainly in the elderly.

Suppurate is to generate pus, to fester.

Suture is a surgical stitch and the material – silk thread, wire or catgut – which holds two surfaces together. It is the surgical uniting of two surfaces by means of stitching.

Squamous carcinoma is an ulcerating malignant tumour which may spread to other parts of the body. On the skin it tends to arise where there has been previous damage, for example, radiation damage, burns or scalds.

You will no doubt meet many other medical terms but this list will give you a good grounding for work with plastic surgery.

Referrals of patients will also be made from dermatology clinics. The word dermatology derives from the Greek 'derma' meaning 'skin'. The dermatologist, therefore, is one who specialises in the skin and its functions and disorders. In the United Kingdom he or she holds a medical degree and is correctly addressed as Doctor.

The number of skin conditions presented to the dermatologist is enormous and the majority of them need not concern the cosmetician. However, there are certain common conditions that are neither infectious nor contagious but merely unsightly, and such cases will be regularly referred for camouflage. Hypopigmentation and hyperpigmentation are the causes of much distress to patients, who are frequently bombarded with such questions as 'is it catching?', 'can't they do something about it?' and so on. Not surprisingly this causes many sufferers to withdraw from society.

Many skin conditions only concern discolouration, with no swelling or distortion to the surface of the skin. For them camouflage is easy, the results being almost miraculous for the patient and most satisfactory for the cosmetician. Sometimes the state of the patient's skin may be poor, with open pores, unnecessary spots or perhaps a dry surface resulting from little or no care being taken of it beyond soap and water. Not only can you improve the appearance with camouflage but you can give advice on proper skin care and cleansing (see Chapter 9, *Care of the skin*). There is little doubt that if your advice is put into practice, the patient's lifestyle will change.

CONDITIONS COMMONLY REFERRED FOR CAMOUFLAGE

Acne is a condition which can leave pitting and unfortunately this is difficult, if not impossible, to disguise with camouflage. It is an inflammatory disorder of the sebaceous glands which results from an excess of sebum production and blockage of the sebaceous gland duct with a plug of keratin, that is, a black head or comedo. It tends to occur from puberty onwards in individuals who are otherwise normal and show no evidence of hormonal abnormalities. A small number of women with acne persisting into their late twenties and thirties have hormonal problems with co-existing menstrual abnormalities, facial hirsutism and hair loss from the scalp. A dermatologist can help with acne and the combined efforts of a dermatologist and a cosmetician can be of great benefit.

Chloasma is characterised by patchy hyperpigmentation of the skin, most usually around the eyes or on the cheeks, occurring occasionally during pregnancy or in those taking the contraceptive pill.

Discoid lupus erythematosis is a patchy inflammatory disorder of the skin occurring mainly on the face and sometimes elsewhere. The lesions may be aggravated by exposure to sunlight and usually heal with scarring. The vast majority of patients with this condition show no evidence of internal disease of the type seen in systemic lupus erythematosis.

Erythema is redness of the skin.

Haemangioma is the abnormal growth of benign tumours of blood vessels.

Leucoderma is hypopigmentation of the skin, with colour being lost in patches.

Naevus is the overall name for the large variety of birthmarks and developmental abnormalities. The commonest involve the melanocyte, for example the melanoctic naevus or mole and the congenital pigmented hairy naevus (bathing trunk naevus). Three of the most common variations of vascular naevus are 1) strawberry naevus, 2) spider naevus and 3) port wine stain.

1) *Strawberry naevus* is the name given to a raised and distorted area, resembling a bunch of strawberries. Most often sited on the face, it is bright pink or red, appears a few days or weeks after birth and usually clears completely by the age of eight. It is very difficult to camouflage.

2) *Spider naevus* has a small central red spot surrounded by several thin blood capillaries on the surface of the skin, the whole of the affected area being probably no more than two centimetres in width. There is no distortion of the skin so it is easily camouflaged.

3) *Port wine stain* is the type of birthmark showing red or purple patches on the skin. Patients with these birthmarks may be referred for camouflage either by a plastic surgeon or a dermatologist, the former being concerned when a request has been made by the patient for removal of the offending mark. In a few cases removal is possible but is often ill advised, especially where there is discolouration but no distortion of the skin. Grafting must necessarily leave scarring which is more difficult to disguise than the stain itself. Camouflage will be suggested as an alternative and excellent results can be obtained.

Psoriasis is a common disorder giving rise to patches (plaques) of salmon pink scaley skin mainly on the elbows and knees but sometimes on the scalp and other parts of the body. It is not infectious.

Rosacea produces a blotchy, flushed appearance on the cheeks and forehead, with papules and pustules. Though distressing for the patient, it is easily camouflaged.

Sebaceous glands are generally attached to the hair follicles, or hair housing. They secrete a fatty substance called sebum which keeps the hair and skin supple and healthy. Over-action of these glands in puberty leads to spots and eruptions on the face. Although not the cause of acne, when the skin is not properly cleansed and where infection sets in, this over-action can be a contributory factor.

Sebum is the fatty substance secreted by the sebaceous glands.

Vitiligo is a condition causing pure white patches to appear on the skin, particularly on the face and hands. It is depigmentation rather than hypopigmentation. Lack of protective pigment leads to a partial sensitivity to sunlight. Most distressing in darker skins, it is easily and effectively camouflaged.

The possibility will arise that once you have become fully established with your camouflage work, you may receive referrals from other branches of the medical profession. Of the numerous possibilities, two particularly spring to mind.

Referrals may come from a **paediatrician,** who specialises in the care of children, or an **endocrinologist,** who specialises in the study of the glandular system. Referrals may include patients suffering complete loss or absence of hair where the grafting of hair-bearing flaps is impossible because no hair-bearing skin is available. Advice might be sought regarding eyebrows and eye-lashes in these cases.

There is no doubt that, as the service grows, so will the expertise of cosmeticians and different types of patient will be referred for help.

12

Training

As yet cosmetic camouflage has not been taught in great depth as a separate subject but has only been briefly touched upon as an adjunct to the wider field of beauty therapy. The challenge to treat it as a specialised subject in its own right has been largely overlooked and indeed, it must be accepted that not all students on beauty courses would be either willing or capable of carrying out such a service.

This book endeavours to bring a greater awareness of what is possible, and to encourage expertise in those who feel they have an affinity with this type of work. Nevertheless, as not everyone is suited to it, training should include exercises which help students to see more clearly whether they would wish to become deeply involved.

Students should be able to understand a little, at least, of how it feels to look 'different' or unacceptable to society at large, so it is reasonable that these feelings should be put to the test while under training. Far better that a student discovers she cannot cope with a traumatic situation before camouflage work is undertaken, than that she should make a patient feel rejected at a later stage. It must be understood that cosmetic camouflage does not in itself offer a glamorous career and its appeal to students may be limited.

For those who are already instructing in this particular field and who may be unsure of how to judge a student's suitability, the following may be helpful.

Students should be put to work in pairs and in turn given the task of applying an ageing make-up to each other, with the object of changing their partner's appearance in as uncomplimentary a way as possible. The knowledge of highlighting and shading can be applied to create lines and shadows which follow the natural lines of tension. Cheeks can be made puffier with the addition of skin plastic, nose putty, latex or wax, as also can noses and overhanging lids. The aim is to produce as natural an appearance as possible,

not one that is theatrical and artificial. A great deal can be learned during this exercise but the most important aspect of it will be the student's reaction when she sees herself with such an unattractive appearance. To see yourself completely changed and looking hideous can be a rather shocking experience but it will help you understand just how deep the feelings of personal revulsion can be when a traumatic change of appearance occurs, and you will glimpse the lack of confidence which would inevitably follow.

It will always be difficult to find models with scarring for a class to practise on, particularly any who are extrovert enough to be used for training purposes. Some schools try to overcome this problem by applying scars on to the students with make-up. This cannot be a satisfactory solution, because the make-up will not be a stable enough base over which to apply the cover creams, remembering that these should be applied directly to scarring.

To some extent this problem can be overcome with other simple exercises. First ask the students to camouflage a specific area of skin on one of their own arms. When complete, the camouflage area must be undetectable. Faults must be matched to the surrounding area and the basic skin colour matched perfectly. An evenly tanned skin is not difficult to match, but fair skinned students will have freckles and uneven marking to simulate.

After completing this exercise satisfactorily, students should then do the same exercise on one another. If the areas chosen to be camouflaged run round the arm, this exercise will be more exacting and difficult to accomplish. The colour change from the back to the front of the arm is considerable and this area is one of the most difficult to camouflage well. Ample time should be allowed for these various tests during training, so that techniques for future work can be well established.

Next each student can cover up an imaginary birthmark on her partner which covers the whole of one cheek, and this extends right up into the lower lid, out beyond the hairline into the scalp, down to the jawline and across to the nose. (See illustration p. 102.)

While there is no actual discolouration to cover, the camouflage will need to be dense enough to cover imaginary hyperpigmentation. If it has been decided that the mark is basically a red one, a pure white cream, or Dermacolor 1742 or D0, or Veil Olive can be used as first coat. If the birthmark is to be one which shows a depth of blue in it, then a first coat of one of the red toners would provide a better finish. In either case, the first coat will need to be set and blotted before the matching basic skin tone is applied on top.

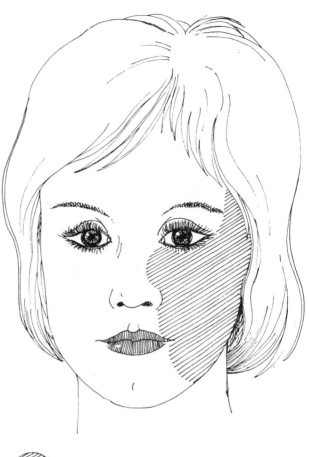

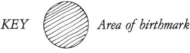 KEY _Area of birthmark_

Covering this type of mark will involve a student in several methods of application. For example: the main area cream will be applied with the finger, but where the application is extended into the hairline, a damp sponge will be the only method of applying the cream without affecting or marking the hair. Application under the lower lid will only be satisfactory when a brush is used – with the model looking up – to enable the cream to be placed right up close to the edge of the eyelid.

This particular exercise will not only familiarise the students with the different methods of application but also make them aware of how it actually feels to wear camouflage. After the camouflage has been judged to have been applied successfully, it can be set, and a

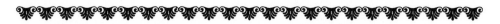

normal make-up applied over it. At the end of this session there should be no evidence of camouflage having been applied and to extend the test further, students could be asked to continue wearing it until the end of the day.

These various methods of training have been tried with success and have not only enabled the instructor to judge the suitability of students for this work, but have also helped the students to see more clearly whether they themselves wish to continue with this work.

Short courses are often available with the various manufacturers of cover creams using their own products, and enquiries about the availability of such courses should be sent to the individual companies.

It is to be hoped that more fully comprehensive training will become more widely available as the need for competent clinical cosmeticians continues to grow.

Skin colour category	Countries	Cover creams within the range of skin matching colour
A	e.g. E and W Europe, N America, S Australia, New Zealand, Norway, Denmark, Canada	*Veil* White, Natural, Medium, Natural-Medium, Tan *Dermacolour* D0, D1, D2, D3, D6, D7 *Covermark* White, Light, Peach *Keromask* White (No. 2), Brown (No. 1), Light (No. 9)
B	e.g. E and W Europe, N America, S Australia, New Zealand, Norway, Denmark, Canada	*Veil* White, Natural, Medium, Natural-Medium, Tan *Dermacolor* D0, D1, D2, D3, D6, D7 *Covermark* White, Light, Peach, Medium *Keromask* White (No. 2), Brown (No. 1), Light (No. 9)
C	e.g. E and W Europe, N America, S Australia, New Zealand, Norway, Denmark, Canada	*Veil* White, Natural, Medium, Natural-Medium, Tan *Dermacolor* D0, D1, D2, D3, D4, D6, D7, D8 *Covermark* White, Light, Peach, Medium *Keromask* White (No. 2), Brown (No. 1), Light (No. 9) *Dermablend* Chroma No. 1 and No. 2
D	e.g. E and W Europe, N America, S Australia, New Zealand, Norway, Denmark, Canada, N India, Pakistan, Bangladesh	*Veil* White, Dark, Natural-Tan, Tan *Dermacolor* D0, D3, D4, D5, D6, D7, D8 *Covermark* White, Medium, Brunette, Rose Dark *Keromask* White (No. 2), Brown (No. 1), Light (No. 9), Medium (No. 10) *Dermablend* Chroma No. 1 and No. 2
E	e.g. E and W Europe, N America, S Australia, New Zealand, Norway, Denmark, Canada, N India, Pakistan, Bangladesh	*Veil* White, Dark, Natural-Tan, Tan, Suntan, Dark No. 3 *Dermacolor* D0, D3, D4, D5, D6, D8, D9 *Covermark* White, Medium, Brunette, Rose Dark *Keromask* White (No. 2), Brown (No. 1), Medium (No. 10) *Dermablend* Chroma No. 2, No. 2A and No. 3
F	e.g. E and W Europe, N America, S Australia, New Zealand, Norway, Canada, N India, Pakistan, Bangladesh, China, Japan, Middle East	*Veil* White, Dark, Suntan, Dark No. 2 and No. 3 *Dermacolor* D0, D4, D5, D8, D9, D10, D18, D19 *Covermark* White, Rose Dark, Dark Brown *Keromask* White (No. 2), Brown (No. 1), Medium (No. 10), Dark (No. 11), Chestnut (No. 7), Yellow (No. 5) *Dermablend* Chroma No. 2, No. 2A and No. 3
G	e.g. India, Pakistan, Bangladesh, China, Japan, Middle East, N American Indians, N Australia, Caribbean, Nigeria, Uganda, Sudan, Zimbabwe, Congo, Tanzania	*Veil* Dark No. 2, Dark No. 3, Brown *Dermacolor* D4, D5, D6, D8, D9, D10, D11, D13, D18, D19, D20, FD *Covermark* No. 1 *Keromask* Dark (No. 11), Chestnut (No. 7), Yellow (No. 5) *Dermablend* Chroma No. 3 and No. 4
H	e.g. S India, Sri Lanka, China, Japan, Middle East, N American Indians, Caribbean, Uganda, Sudan, Zimbabwe, Congo, Tanzania, Malawi, Zaire, Mozambique	*Veil* Brown *Dermacolor* D5, D10, D11, D13, D18, D19, D20 *Covermark* No. 1, No. 8 *Keromask* Dark (No. 11), Chestnut (No. 7), Yellow (No. 5), Rose (No. 4) *Dermablend* Chroma No. 4, No. 5 and No. 6
I	e.g. S India, Sri Lanka, Middle East, Caribbean, Uganda, Sudan, Zimbabwe, Tanzania, Zambia, Malawi, Zaire, Mozambique	*Dermacolor* D14, D15, D16, D17 *Covermark* No. 8, No. 3 *Keromask* Chestnut (No. 7), Umber (No. 8), Rose (No. 4) *Dermablend* Chroma No. 6 and No. 7
J	e.g. Uganda, Sudan, Zimbabwe, Tanzania, Zambia, Malawi, Zaire, Mozambique	*Dermacolor* D15, D16, D17, D17A, D40 *Keromask* Chestnut (No. 7), Umber (No. 8), Rose (No. 4), Black (No. 6)

Note Dermacolor D0 and Veil and Keromask White are included in the colour matching shades in categories A–F as they can be used to lighten any of the other colours as necessary.

Index